MEN, MOLDS, AND HISTORY

MEN,
MOLDS,
AND
HISTORY

FELIX MARTI-IBAÑEZ, M.D.

Professor and Director of the Department of the History of Medicine,
New York Medical College,
Flower and Fifth Avenue Hospitals, New York, N. Y.

Editor-in-Chief of MD Medical Newsmagazine

MD PUBLICATIONS, INC.
New York

Henry Welch, Ph.D., Director
Division of Antibiotics
Food and Drug Administration
Washington, D. C.

My dear Henry:

To dedicate this book to you affords me great honor and much pleasure. It is a handful of articles and addresses on philosophical and historical aspects of antibiotics, written or delivered on various occasions when you were present, either in person, as one of the foremost scientific figures in this field, or in spirit guiding me always with your wisdom.

My cultural interest in the field of research and clinical application of antibiotics extends back many years. I was attracted to this dynamic branch of modern medicine by its historical importance in the evolution of therapeutics, by the drama that attended the discovery and clinical application of antibiotics, and by the multiple facets and consequences of their introduction in modern medicine. But only when I became acquainted with you personally—and we embarked together on the vast project of compiling a corpus doctrinalis *on antibiotic medicine that would create an intellectual, academic and journalistic frame to encompass the enormous mass of knowledge accumulated in this field—did I dare, like a swimmer short of breath but filled with great enthusiasm, to dive into the deep, shoreless ocean of antibiotic medicine, of which you are an experienced and expert navigator.*

To your many gifts as an imaginative scientific investigator and as an indefatigable organizer with a flair for creating research teams and welding them together with the fire of your enthusiasm, is added the gift of the born teacher. This is confirmed by both your spoken words, with which you can like the artist with his crayon so flowingly and limpidly delineate the most complex scientific problems, and your written words, those polished mirrors that always reflect the honest purity of your scientific truth. It was indeed a happy coincidence, hearalding your future career, that you should receive your Master's Degree from Brown University in 1928, the same year as the discovery of penicillin.

It has been my good fortune to have shared with you some ten years of toil in creating an international antibiotic discipline through symposia, books, journals, scientific papers, and editorials. I have learned much by working at your side. I have also had the opportunity in those years of intellectual and spiritual relationship to observe and appreciate the fine human qualities concealed beneath your austere exterior of the man of science, qualities that relieve this self-imposed austerity, just as merry splashes of gentian violet on the scientist's smock relieve its forbidding aseptic whiteness.

The humanistic nature of your work, your vigorous determination to contribute at the expense of your leisure and pleasure to the accelerated progress of antibiotic medicine, your proverbial frankness and sincerity, your scientific and intellectual probity—all these combine to make you the prototype of the "modern" savant, "modern" because your impassioned concentration on one single, though ever-expanding, field of research and your encyclopedic knowledge of it are happily combined with a vast range of human interests and diversions, from amusing chit-chat to serious golf. And as if this were not enough, there is also the honey of your genial sense of humor, unknown to many because you discretely keep it out of easy reach, like the dates atop the palm tree, reserving it only for special occasions and certain persons.

Because I have watched you painstakingly chiseling, day after day, year after year, an important scientific block of the medicine of our time, I dedicate to you these essays, a part of my modest literary harvest on antibiotics. The rest of which is included in my book Centaur: Essays on the History of Medical Ideas *and in the section on antibiotic medicine in my forthcoming history of medicine entitled* The Fabric of Medicine. *In these two books I have outlined in greater detail, with names and dates, the history of antibiotics, which from a mere trickling of water of humble empiric origin has grown into a majestic Amazon whose mighty flow has changed the face of modern medicine before emptying into the ocean of History.*

In this book I have set down some of the concepts and ideas, born very often during conversations with you or revolving around events planned and organized together while we were seated in offices as busy as beehives or in the white silence of laboratories in New York and Washington, while strolling through polychrome parks on the banks of the Seine in Paris, watching the churling muddy waters

*of the Thames in London, or zooming in enormous birds of silver
across the Atlantic.*

    *On all these occasions, in exchange for my dreams as a historian
you always gave me the golden nuggets of your wisdom. This book
is my tribute to your generosity and to your untiring labors with
pen and word, forever wielded like oars toward new shores in the
vast realm of Antibiotic Medicine.*

FELIX MARTI-IBAÑEZ, M.D.

*September, 1958
New York, N. Y.*

The following is a list of the chapters in this book with their original sources of publication.

HISTORICAL PERSPECTIVES OF ANTIBIOTICS, copyrighted in *Antibiotics & Chemotherapy 3*:1187, 1953. Also delivered at the First Annual Symposium on Antibiotics, Washington, D. C., 1953.

THE PHILOSOPHIC IMPACT OF ANTIBIOTICS ON CLINICAL MEDICINE, copyrighted in *Antibiotic Medicine 1*:398, 1955. Also delivered at the Second Annual Symposium on Antibiotics, Washington, D. C., 1954.

THE NEXT HALF CENTURY IN ANTIBIOTIC MEDICINE AND ITS EFFECT ON THE HISTORY OF THE CLINICAL CASE HISTORY, copyrighted in *Antibiotic Medicine & Clinical Therapy 3*:50, 1956. Also delivered at the Third Annual Symposium on Antibiotics, Washington, D. C., 1955.

ANTIBIOTICS TODAY AND THE MEDICINE OF THE FUTURE, copyrighted in *Antibiotics & Chemotherapy 5* (supp. 1):21, 1955. Also delivered at the International Symposium on Antibiotics, New York City, 1954.

IN QUEST OF THE BROAD SPECTRUM, copyrighted in *International Record of Medicine and General Practice Clinics 168*:103, 1955.

ANTIBIOTICS AND THE PROBLEM OF MEDICAL COMMUNICATION, copyrighted in *Antibiotic Medicine & Clinical Therapy 4*:524, 1957. Also delivered at the Fourth Annual Symposium on Antibiotics, Washington, D. C., 1956.

WORDS AND RESEARCH, copyrighted in *Antibiotic Medicine & Clinical Therapy 4*:740, 1957. Also delivered at the Fifth Annual Symposium on Antibiotics, Washington, D. C., 1957.

THE MEANING OF GREATNESS, copyrighted in *International Record of Medicine and General Practice Clinics 168*:199, 1955.

ON TREATING THE WHOLE PATIENT, copyrighted in *Antibiotic Medicine 1*:247, 1955.

ON THE ART OF TRANSLATION AND THE SCIENCE OF ANTIBIOTICS, copyrighted in *Principios y Practica de la Terapia Antibiotica,* New York, Medical Encyclopedia, Inc., 1955, p. xi.

CONTENTS

MEN, MOLDS, AND HISTORY

HISTORICAL PERSPECTIVES OF ANTIBIOTICS

THE ERA OF ANTIBIOTICS

It is a great honor to be given the opportunity to address and welcome, as International Editor of *Antibiotics & Chemotherapy,* such a distinguished group of scientists; but I wish to emphasize that I have come here with that "student's spirit" of listening and learning recommended by my teacher, Ramón y Cajal. This is perhaps the first time that research workers, clinicians, professors, chemists, and bacteriologists have come together with one single purpose: to study antibiotics from different viewpoints. That is why this meeting is of great historical importance.

In the history of medicine there is perhaps no other event as revolutionary as the discovery of antibiotics. What we now call the "Antibiotic Era"—an era that began in 1939–1940 with the work of Dubos, Chain and Florey, and Waksman—was preceded by Pasteur's and Koch's bacteriologic discoveries, Lister's prophylactic chemotherapy for septic wounds, and scientific chemotherapy (originally started as selective chromotherapy), with which Ehrlich opened the gates to modern therapeutics. Since the first clinical application of antibiotics twelve years ago, our way of thinking in medicine, our scientific semantics, and especially our philosophic views concerning the art of healing have changed radically; and yet we have experienced only the beginning of the influence of these drugs on medicine.

Delivered at the First Annual Symposium on Antibiotics, Washington, D. C., October 28–30, 1953.

At the beginning of the nineteenth century, therapeutics, as Sir Francis Fraser pointed out, had not changed in fifteen hundred years. Before Hippocrates, it was believed that illness was produced by demoniac forces against which only magical rituals and exorcism were of any avail. At the dawn of the last century, disease was still considered to be the result of a "foreign body" that might be expelled by means of purgatives, diuretics, emetics, diaphoretics, and bloodletting. Auscultation and percussion soon after enriched the sources of diagnosis. But the arsenal of therapeutics remained untapped. Only at the end of the nineteenth century did we see, with the introduction of synthetic antipyretics, thyroid extracts, and vaccines, the crystallization of new allopathic, immunobiologic, and endocrinologic therapeutics, later followed by the discoveries of vitaminology. But nothing revolutionized therapeutics as much as the introduction of antibiotics in our century, and not so much because of their spectacular effects as because they represented a new concept of the art of healing.

Just as in the phylogenic evolution of an animal organism the humoral and nervous correlations precede the formation of the organized nervous system, and the hormones precede the appearance of the endocrine glands, so in medicine many drugs were used empirically for centuries before scientific knowledge was crystallized into a doctrinal corpus.

We know that antibiotics were probably the active principle of the ancient Chinese soy-flour poultices, of the "yeast of sweet beer" mentioned in the Ebers Papyrus (1500 B.C.), of the *cuxum* fungi used by the ancient Mayans (the fungi discussed by Pliny the Elder, A.D. first century), of medieval cataplasms, and of the *unguentum sympatheticum* that John Parkinson, the King's apothecary (1567–1650), made with *muscus ex cranio humano* or "mosse upon dead men's sculles." We also know that Tyndall's experiments, described in his *Essays on the Floating Matter of the Air in Relation to Putrefaction and Infection* (1881), represented the historical prelude to the discovery of antibiotics, although Tyndall did not lift but barely brushed the veil that hid the mystery.

INDIVIDUAL AND TEAM WORK

The discovery of penicillin by Fleming was the work of one man. Science in the past often progressed by the impact of chance or coincidence upon the brilliant insight of genius. But later discoveries, especially the discovery of the whole roster of antibiotics, have been the collective work of organized teams of researchers. If penicillin was discovered through a fortunate stroke of luck interpreted by a well-disciplined scientific mind, the newer antibiotics are the result of "organized chance," of systematic investigation in which luck is "created" by a team of scientists who veritably squeeze from the earth bactericidal powers that, like sleeping beauties, had lain dormant for thousands of years.

THE UNIVERSALITY OF ANTIBIOTICS

In past centuries the discovery of a new drug with therapeutic powers was always wrapped in mystery. From the medieval alchemists to the German apothecaries of the last century, the discovery of a drug was a source of legitimate but dangerous individual and national pride. That patriotic vanity made it difficult for the new drug to become universally recognized. Antibiotics have done more than any other drug in history to universalize medicine. The search for an antibiotic substance begins by obtaining samples of earth from the four corners of the planet. Today, a clod of earth picked up in some field in the Orient by an Australian pilot and developed by North American microbiologists may be applied in the form of a new antibiotic by a European physician to save the life of a Latin-American patient. Can one ask for a greater therapeutic universality?

We can go even further. We can say that work in antibiotics is more international than in any other area of science, because its principal source is in the earth, and it is difficult, if not impossible, to claim that what Nature meant to belong to the entire world and to serve all ailing mankind is the exclusive property of one scientist or one country. Antibiotics have also made possible the great international campaigns of the World Health Organization for the prevention and cure of many of the ancient scourges of mankind.

CIVIL WARS BETWEEN MICROBES

Since antibiotics go back in time to the dawn of history and are universal in space, we should not be surprised that they have shaken contemporary scientific thought to its very foundations and upset many of our philosophic taboos. Medical interest was suddenly focused on the earth as a source of therapeutically valuable substances, which, although previously known, had never crossed the barrier separating theoretical science from practical applied medicine. Only recently did antibiotics cease to be a riddle to science and become a problem in applied technology.

Man's sustenance comes directly or indirectly from the earth; the correlation between the different soils of the world and the health of the various nations dependent upon them is well known. Society, like any well-constructed building, does not rise from the surface of the ground but from the depths of the earth itself. The phenomenon known as *antagonism* or *antibiosis* of the soil had been known for more than a century, and so had the bacterial capacity of the soil to produce antimicrobic substances; but the idea of applying those properties chemotherapeutically was both new and revolutionary.

Until a few years ago, the fight among microbes was considered a substantiation of the Darwinian notion of the struggle for life, and their substances were called "lysins," "toxins," or "bacteriolysins." Today they are called antibiotics. Only in the last dozen years have we availed ourselves widely of what was long studied only as a rarity of nature and then only by a few laboratory hermits. But man, after discovering that he could fight disease by producing it in miniature with vaccines (just as a large fire may be neutralized by a smaller fire), has finally learned to benefit by the incessant civil wars waged by microbes and to introduce into the ranks of enemy microbes "fifth columns" of friendly microbes capable of both destroying the enemy and rescuing the patient.

ACTIVITY AND TOXICITY OF ANTIBIOTICS

To the knowledge that the earth and the sea are inexhaustible sources of antibiotics—research workers are exploring fifty thousand known species of molds in their search for new antibiotics—has been added a revision of the classic pharmacologic concepts whereby greatly toxic drugs may be turned into therapeutic agents.

In the past, when a drug was found to be toxic to the human organism, it was replaced by others less toxic but also less active. Antibiotic research has helped dissipate that terror of toxic drugs. Today we know that the therapeutic activity of a drug is often parallel to its toxicity; our new philosophic outlook is not to discard an antibiotic because it is toxic, but to find a way of reducing its toxicity or to search for a less toxic derivative that is equally effective.

INTERFERENCE WITH MICROBE METABOLISM

Antibiotics have also helped us to look at the problem of microbe activity in a new light: we know that not all microbes are our enemies, and that life in general is made possible by the activity of bacteria. The old post-Pasteurian concept that almost all microbes are pathogenic agents, and as such undesirable, has been replaced by the idea that they quite often are part of symbiotic processes necessary to human life. Man has learned to use for his own benefit the antibiotic substances produced by microbes to destroy their competitors for the food of the soil.

This medical curiosity about the life of microbes has led research workers to look into the reason for their therapeutic effects. Investigators have penetrated the mysteries of the interrelationships among microbes and have provoked, as often happens with chemotherapeutic agents, "deficiency diseases" in microbes—after the manner of avitaminosis, if I may be permitted the analogy.

In short, the attempt has been to interfere with microbe metabolism, to throw a "monkey wrench" into the subtle and complex metabolic machinery of microbes, and, by paralyzing it or breaking it up, to end its pathogenic effects in man, thereby establishing the anti-infectious medicine of the future. The discovery of antibiotic substances in nature has stimulated a desire to synthesize them chemically and to seek out the enzymatic activities in which their secret may lie. And so the objective of the second stage of the Antibiotic Era may be twofold: metabolic interference with the life of microbes and enzymatic research.

The problem is now centered not so much on increasing the number of antibiotics—of the three hundred known to us only about a score can be used clinically—as on stimulating their qualitative selectivity and attenuating their toxicity by synthesizing new derivatives to help fight the ever-growing problem of microbial resistance to antibiotics. In the struggle between man and microbes, the latter defend themselves by developing a growing resistance to weapons that are lethal at the outset but to which they may eventually become accustomed. The goal of the research worker, therefore, is to forge new weapons against each new shield contrived by the bacteria, to create antibiotic agents that, like modern Attilas, will destroy every single stronghold put up by the microbes.

ANTIBIOTICS IN THE CLINIC AND LABORATORY DIAGNOSIS

Antibiotics have been unjustly accused of encouraging physicians to treat the disease first and to diagnose it later. It has been said that the physician stuffs his patient with antibiotics and then makes his diagnosis by a process of elimination, depending on the effectiveness or ineffectiveness of certain antibiotics. I do not agree. The practicing physician was never so engrossed in fine and subtle diagnostic problems in infections as he has been since the advent of antibiotics.

From time immemorial a dichotomy has existed between the clinician and the laboratory technician. For the laboratory researcher, the practicing physician was only a routinized professional dulled by his daily tasks; for the physician, the laboratory man was a dreamy visionary who had lost contact with reality, who lived in an ivory tower with his crucibles and looked at the world through the eyepiece of his microscope. Antibiotics have brought the physician and the investigator together. Today, the physician is interested in the problems of laboratory diagnoses, and the laboratory man has learned to temper his work with mold cultures with a spirit of human concern for their effects on the patient, which are now brought to his attention by the physician's reports.

Furthermore, antibiotics have enlarged research teams to include the clinical pathologist—today the intermediary between the laboratory and the clinic—whose work becomes more indispensable all the time, the microbiologist, the botanist, the chemical engineer, and many other scientists who were hitherto barred from the domain of the laboratory technician.

THE SCIENTIFIC SUBCONSCIOUS OF A COUNTRY

Among those who have contributed the most to the antibiotic crusade are the research workers of pharmaceutical companies. They often are the anonymous heroes of the crusade. To them I render special homage. If I may be permitted a psychiatric simile, I would say that universities and hospitals represent the scientific consciousness of a nation, while the laboratories of pharmaceutical companies represent its scientific subconscious. Those who represent scientific consciousness are often in the light; but the research workers of the pharmaceutical industry labor in the quiet but fertile shadows that mark the subconscious. And just as the authentic truth about man emanates from the subconscious in the form of dreams and inspirations, so does many a great truth responsible for notable progress in science emanate from this scientific subconscious of a nation represented by pharmaceutical laboratories. And just as in an iceberg the most important part is invisible under the water, so in the field of antibiotics the most important part is constituted by the invisible research workers in the pharmaceutical industry, who have anonymously contributed some of the most notable discoveries in this field.

ANTIBIOTICS AS INDUSTRIAL OR GOVERNMENT PROPERTY

It has often been debated whether antibiotics should be the property of national governments and be distributed by them, or whether they should continue to belong to the pharmaceutical companies that discover them. To ask such a question is the same as asking whether the blue of the sky should belong only to the poets who extol it. I believe that free competition among pharmaceutical companies has been responsible for the fantastic progress in antibiotic medicine in the last few years. The logical step would be for such companies, guided by their governments and the ideal to serve man's welfare, to ensure that the greatest number of patients of all races, religions, nationalities, and social positions would be aided by their discoveries under the best possible conditions. This would require harmonious co-operation among the various pharmaceutical companies. Should such co-operation be developed, antibiotics will truly deserve the name "miracle drug." I am one of those optimists who prophesies that this will come about.

ANTIBIOTICS AND MEDICAL JOURNALISM

In conclusion, I would like to mention the effect of antibiotics on medical journals and the teaching of medicine.

As a means of spreading scientific progress, we must especially emphasize the service rendered by medical journalism to the new antibiotic medicine. One of the great ideals of William Osler was to bring physicians of different specialties together in the pages of medical journals, as if in a club hall with a glowing fireplace and comfortable armchairs. There are already unbiased journals that give space to the discoveries of both the research worker and the clinician and to their different and often, especially in the field of antibiotics, contradictory viewpoints. In all my years of medical writing, I have never known medical journals to contribute so prolifically to a medical cause as they do to antibiotics. In Japan and in the United States, certain journals dedicated exclusively to antibiotics and chemotherapy publish complete articles on this *nuova scienza,* thus converting their pages into veritable reference documents. These journals are true university chairs on paper, and from them one can learn painlessly the principles of this new science. Never before have journals deserved so much the term used by Sir Francis Bacon in his *New Atlantis*—"merchants of light."

UNIVERSITY CHAIRS OF ANTIBIOTIC MEDICINE

As important as the effect on medical journals is the revolution that antibiotics have brought about in the teaching of medicine. A school of medicine, if it wishes to accomplish its historical mission, must be a center of research, teaching, and clinical work. At schools of medicine we learn the art of healing; we become practicing physicians, research workers, or teachers. Antibiotics have converted modern medical textbooks into historical curios. The medical student today already discards as Hippocratic anachronisms notions that were accepted only ten years ago: the almost mathematical fever cycles of certain infections, the crisis in pneumonia, the epidemiology of certain tropical diseases, and, of course, the therapy of venereal diseases and infections in general. For the first time in the history of medicine a new therapeutic system has torn down, like Samson, the classic axioms in medicine that held up the temple of contemporary medical knowledge. It has revolutionized the concept of diagnosis, prognosis, and epidemiology of the majority of infections and, of course, their prophylaxis and treatment. With time, even the biologic cycles of causal germs will change as the latter develop resistance against antibiotics and their virulence grows stronger or weaker, thus changing even the natural history of many illnesses.

This means that in the laboratory and in the hospital there is rapidly taking shape a totally new doctrinal *Corpus,* which already encompasses sections of the laboratory, clinic, pathology, microbiology, hygiene and public health, sanitary engineering, and even medical sociology. For as people live longer, there will be an increasing percentage of old people who will cease to constitute a geriatric problem and will become a question of political sociology. That is why it is imperative—and I take this opportunity to launch the idea publicly for the first time—that Chairs of Antibiotic Medicine be created. And when these Chairs are created throughout the nation, it is my hope that the United States will encourage other countries to enrich the teaching of medicine with professorships of antibiotic medicine. This very symposium might do further pioneer work by drawing up a proposal urging the creation of such university chairs. Not only will these Chairs of Antibiotic Medicine be instruments of education, but they will also serve as centers of antibiotic research and study. Further research, for example, in the development of synergistic combinations, the antibiotic therapy of virus diseases, the solution to the problem of germ resistance, and the treatment of fungus diseases may stem from these new centers of research.

On October 27, 1953, the medical world commemorated the four-hundredth anniversary of the death of one of the greatest figures in medical history, the Spaniard Miguel Servet, discoverer of pulmonary circulation, who was burnt at the stake in Geneva because he believed in and fought for freedom of thought and scientific truth.

Miguel Servet said that the mission of the man of science is to search for Truth. Gentlemen, because you were preoccupied by the search for Truth you became occupied in research for Science. May you be guided in your search for scientific truth by the same spirit that four centuries ago inspired the life and death of a great man of science.

THE PHILOSOPHIC IMPACT OF
ANTIBIOTICS ON CLINICAL MEDICINE

THE TWO OCCUPATIONS OF MAN

Perhaps man's two most engrossing occupations are to remember and to dream: to recall the past in his memories and to anticipate the future in his hopes. "To live with the full consciousness of living," said the great Spanish writer Pérez Galdós, "is to recall the past and to dream of the future."

In no other scientific field as in medicine can both occupations be more fruitful. By looking back, the physician benefits from the signposts on the path traced by the evolution of medical thought, and by peering into the future, he can steer his endeavors along the routes blazed on the horizon. To glance backward through the history of medicine is not only to uncover a multitude of points of departure from which thought can take great leaps forward, but also to harvest the lesson of past errors and thus avoid repeating them. To look ahead is to gaze on a constellation of stars which, although unreachable, will nevertheless help, as they help the navigator, to set the course toward port.

THE DUTY TO PHILOSOPHIZE

If we disregard the historical roots of the age-old empirical use of molds and fungi, antibiotic medicine can be said to be a scientific discipline almost without a past. It is all present and future. From the memorable day in 1928 when a humble spore of *Penicillium notatum*

Delivered at the Second Annual Symposium on Antibiotics, Washington, D. C., October 25–29, 1954.

descended from the gray, smoky skies of the Borough of Paddington onto the culture of *Staphylococcus aureus* with which Alexander Fleming was working, until the present day when the production of antibiotics runs into millions of dollars, there have elapsed twenty-eight years, yet this quarter of a century is but a flick of the eyelash in the lifetime of history.

Perhaps it is because of this lack of a deep-rooted past, which always helps us face the future with confidence, that there are still so many doubts and uncertainties in the field of antibiotics. That is why this dissertation will be an act of *pre*occupation, one of man's noblest tasks, since *pre*occupation always precedes occupation. The truly civilized man is the one who is capable of being preoccupied and of being so without pessimism, accepting the universe and history as they are, and having no other aim than that of making of his preoccupation a fruitful act leading to creation and progress.

Of course, there are sterile preoccupations, like those that impelled men in the Middle Ages to keep watch from the battlements for the dreaded arrival of the scarlet dawn that supposedly would announce the final judgment, or like those that today bedevil all who fear for the future of mankind because of the atomic menace. But our preoccupation with the future of antibiotic medicine is healthy, because it expresses our double desire for scientific perfection and for the humanitarian expansion of our discipline.

The horoscope of the future is written in the present, and its tapestry is woven with the threads of modern medical knowledge. Therefore, to place the many-colored canvas of antibiotic medicine on an imaginary easel today is to anticipate its future. And that is what I wish to do on this occasion, that is, to follow Hans Selye's advice and distinguish between the two royal roads of progress in medicine: that which follows the technical path signifying the search for knowledge, and that which follows the philosophic path signifying the search for wisdom. Both paths merge forever when our zeal leads us to "a better understanding of Nature and a fundamental evaluation of our discoveries."

It is fitting therefore that we pause at this point to reassess philosophically the progress already made by antibiotic medicine and to trace the areas still to be crossed. In barely twenty-five years antibiotics have revolutionized the three facets—practice, research, teaching—of modern medicine. The physician today treats infections with methods radically different from those he used at the outset of his career; if he is a research worker, he investigates horizons he did not even dream of in the classroom; if he is a teacher, he has witnessed with his own eyes the changes produced by antibiotics in the natural history of infections.

At this point let us briefly review the philosophic impact of antibiotics on modern medicine. And let us not be afraid of the word "philosophic." Webster has defined philosophy abstractly as a code of individual conduct: "Philosophy is a body of principles of general conceptions subject to a determined branch of knowledge." And further: "A personal, integrated and consistent attitude toward life or reality or toward certain phases of these, especially if such an attitude is expressed in beliefs or in principles of conduct." If we ponder these definitions for a moment, we shall realize that the physician is continuously indulging in philosophy without being aware of it, just as Molière's "would-be gentleman" spoke in prose without realizing it.

Let us not forget the great historical duties of the physician: *to heal* by using the what (the drug) and the how (his knowledge); *to contribute to the progress of civilization* by applying his knowledge and experience; *to foresee certain events,* such as the course of diseases or epidemics, which makes him a prophet of the individual and collective biologic history of man; and, finally, *to organize human life* by improving man's housing, clothes, food, and habits. The physician must be able to philosophize in order to fulfill these duties and, ultimately, to place the cornerstone of man's historical destiny.

REASSESSMENT OF MEDICAL FOLKLORE

Medical folklore has undergone a historical evolution, but its directing forces are still the same. Assyrian healers before Christ attempted to expel disease from the body by means of exorcism: they thought they could drive malignant spirits away by producing terror or ecstasy in the patient. This technique was employed century after century up to Mesmer, Bouillaud, and the period of "vampirism" in French medicine, when on the flimsiest therapeutic pretext patients were bled to death. Parallel to this trend there developed the use of medicinal plants, based on the idea that God had created each plant with specific curative powers for each disease. Quinine, ipecacuanha, and digitalis were among the various plants used empirically for many years before they were added to the arsenal of medicine.

Medicine as an art has existed from the beginning of civilization. In the seventh century before Christ—a century of prodigious importance in the progress of mankind—the Ionian Greek philosophers created medical science. They introduced, as a basis for the art and the practice of medicine, scientific knowledge incorporated into two sciences: *physiology* in its broadest sense, that is, physiopathology, and *clinical medicine.* But the empirical use of various substances, such as antibiotics, for curative purposes came considerably earlier.

The era of antibiotics, ushered in by the discovery of penicillin through a fortuitous accident, has led us to reassess medical folklore. Elsewhere I have discussed how antibiotics forced even the most materialistic physicians to meditate on the value of history—that history without which nothing in life has any meaning.

Today scientific interest focuses on the soil of our planet as a source of substances with possible therapeutic value. Many of these substances were known previously but had never been used on a scientific level. Man's sustenance comes directly or indirectly from the earth, and the relationship existing between the earth and the health of those dwelling on it is a point of common knowledge. Human society, like a building, is not founded on ground level but well below the surface, in the bowels of the earth.

The phenomenon of microbial antagonism, or antibiosis, as well as the capacity of bacteria for producing antimicrobial substances, has been known for more than a century, but the idea of applying such properties chemotherapeutically is as new as it is revolutionary. The constant war of the microbes was considered for many years as part of the Darwinian concept of the struggle for existence, and what we call antibiotics were designated as "lysins," "toxins," or "bacteriolysins." Only in the last fourteen years have we made practical use of something that for hundreds of years was studied simply as a rarity of nature.

This inexhaustible reservoir of antibiotics to be found on our planet (it already includes the sea), containing more than fifty thousand known kinds of molds, has caused the scientist to feel irresistibly drawn to the fabulous book of medical folklore, which brims over with legendary remedies that science today is translating into therapeutic realities in the form of antibiotics.

Antibiotics were not discovered in the past because the philosophic idea of "antibiosis" and the concept of the antibiotic powers of nature were not developed until Vuillemin.

ANTIBIOTICS AND THE PHILOSOPHIC NATURE OF DISEASE

Antibiotics have revolutionized the clinical concept of disease held by the physician in our time.

In history there have been two great philosophic concepts of disease: the Hippocratic *nosos,* or disease as the sickness of an *individual,* the becoming ill of a human being, and the *species morbosa* of Sydenham, the basis of which was the view of *general* natural processes deriving from botany. Hippocrates frequently based his clinical descriptions on the observation of a *single* diseased person, while

Sydenham based his on the study of many cases. What Galileo did for physics when he reduced the complexity of the motions of nature to rectilinear and circular movements, Sydenham did for pathology.

In opposition to Sydenham's concept there has arisen in our time an etiologic nosology (*etiology,* let us not forget, comes from the Greek *aitia* meaning "cause"), that is to say, causal thought in medicine, supported by the introduction of antibiotics.

The current etiologic imperative to create a true "bacteriologic clinic" and a "clinical pharmacology" has caused the disintegration of the classic anatomopathologic school. Clinical workers of the last century, for example, erected a vast descriptive scaffolding with their picture of pulmonary congestions. The bacteriologist of today does not understand this picture and has dismantled it and replaced it with the study of the causal microbe.

On the other hand, antibiotics have forced the physician to focus his attention upon the *specific* bacteriologic problem of each disease, thus showing that the *localization* of a germ is what partially determines the resultant lesion. For the physician of twenty years ago, a pneumococcic infection was a pathologic entity that could be rigidly catalogued. The physician of today knows that pneumococcus may cause, depending on its organic location, a pneumonia or a meningitis. In either case bacteriologic specificity dictates the necessary specificity of the treatment.

The concept of the nature of disease held by the physician of today has been notably influenced by the change in therapeutics brought about by the use of antibiotics. If twenty-five years ago it was essential to develop a clinical or anatomopathologic nosology, today it is indispensable to establish an etiologic nosology. The study of the causal germ and its natural history is today as important for an exact diagnosis and an effective therapy as it was years ago to understand thoroughly the configuration of the pathologic lesion.

The problem of the nature of disease, especially of infections, began to be solved as soon as the physician understood that there can be no disease without a patient to harbor it, just as there can be no mind without a brain to house it.

Man is the product of three factors: his genetic origin, his environment—physical, biologic, and mental—and the use he makes of his free will. Yet man's body, considered from a thermodynamic point of view, is a self-adapting, self-maintaining, self-repairing, and self-reproducing physiochemical machine "blueprinted" at the moment of conception. The forces of stress cause this machine to react in different ways, for some men are like flimsy shacks built on sand while others are like fortresses built on rock.

This concept has caused the modern clinical research scientist, who is influenced by the use of antibiotics, to favor a science based on the study of physiopathology. Modern physiology itself is based on the study of pathology, while chemotherapy is based on the study of the pathologic process of infection. There is nothing more physiologic than the pathologic. That which is pathologic is not something strange added to a personality, but rather the reverse of the physiologic personality. Pathologic accidents are accelerated phases of life's essential physiologic process—the inexorable progress toward death.

In contrast to Galenic teleologic physiology, the characteristics of modern physiology are: to study the relationship between organs and not the intrinsic substance of these organs per se; to replace classic qualitative descriptions with exact quantitative measurements; to establish the existing differences and tensions between the form and function of the organs; and to ignore willfully the teleologic object of the viscera.

As a new concept of disease developed, this modern physiology replaced the Assyrian concept of disease as a divine punishment, as well as the Greek concept of disease as a contamination or an impurity. It re-established the idea of disease as dissymmetry (already entertained by the Greeks, for almost everything in modern civilization has its roots in classical Greece), that is, the disturbance of the *symmetron,* which, as Alcmæon of Croton claimed, is the health of man. Disease is the lack of harmony in the *physis* of the patient. Present-day physiopathology is based on functional disturbance caused by dissymmetry and on a "natural" curative effort that this deviation from the norm or *metron* brings with it.*

THE REVINDICATION OF DISEASE AS A GENERIC PROCESS

The use of antibiotics has forced the physician to face a series of antinomies encountered in his daily practice. Among these contradictions is the one raised by the patient as *nature* and as an *individual,* a *biologic entity* and a *conscious being* endowed with free will. Another is the obligation to distinguish between the need for a diagnosis and the imperative duty to apply treatment: *to know* and *to cure,* the cognitive and the operative processes. To these must be added the necessity of differentiating between the individual and society, between the patient as a Robinson Crusoe isolated on the

---

* It is not surprising that certain medical conceptions today are still as they were in the time of Homer. The present-day dichotomy between "scientific" medicine and "psychologic" medicine is the same as that of the pre-Christian era of Hippocratic Greece, when Hippocrates' human, naturalistic, and scientific medicine existed side by side with the "divine" medicine based on the miracles of the Asclepiades.

       MEN, MOLDS, AND HISTORY

inaccessible island of his pain and the patient as an entity embodying the society and culture to which he belongs.

The physician must face both these generic and individual aspects: in treating each patient he must know how to differentiate between *the* disease and the *patient's* disease, the *generic* disturbance studied in books and the *particular* ailment encountered at the patient's bedside. Infections offer the best opportunity to appreciate this dramatic contrast between the patient as an individual and the patient as a dramatic theatre in which the infection is acting itself out. For the physician of Sydenham's time the essential task was to treat *diseases,* to discover the characteristic symptoms of a particular infection and combat it with the limited resources then available. In reaction to this abstract and generic medicine, the modern physician since the beginning of our century has returned to the original Hippocratic art of treating *patients.*

The introduction of antibiotics, however, has somewhat restrained the tendency to see in a patient only the individual case and has, in a way, been responsible for acceptance of him as an example of a generic infection. Historically, the generic is once more on a par with the singular. The philosophic reason for this is that in order to use an antibiotic with therapeutic success, it is necessary to make not only a clinical study of the patient, but also a series of laboratory tests to determine *the characteristics of his particular sickness as a representative case of a generic disease.* The clinic individualizes the patient; the laboratory depersonalizes him. On his hospital bed the patient is a suffering human being; in the laboratory, on the culture plate, in the in vitro reaction, in the test tube, the patient, represented by the specimens obtained from him, is only an abstract expression of a generic disease.

The modern physician, in order to cure an infection, must know not only *how* but also *when* to administer an antibiotic; when he resorts to a series of laboratory procedures, analyses, culture tests, and assays in vivo and in vitro, he is really checking the results of his clinical observations with those of laboratory tests. Thus, the patient becomes *one case* of a certain generic infection. The physician must then make a hurried but accurate synthesis to ascertain which antibiotic should be administered, when and how it should be administered, and when treatment should be interrupted.

This is how antibiotic medicine has forced a philosophic reassessment in modern medicine of the art of healing, reconciling the "to know" (diagnosis) with the "to cure" (therapy), the personal with the generic. A harmonious synthesis of the clinic and the laboratory is effected by the necessity of making antibiotic medicine into a science as practical as it is exact.

Research in antibiotics has given rise to a new concept of the toxicity of the drugs used as therapeutic agents. In the past it was enough to discover that a drug was toxic to human tissue for it to be discarded and replaced by another drug less toxic but also less active. Antibiotics have helped to dispel the terror that toxic drugs formerly inspired. Today we know that in many cases the pharmacologic activity of a drug is in a way parallel to its toxicity, but the philosophic outlook has changed. Now, instead of discarding an antibiotic because of its great toxicity, we investigate the possibility of making it less toxic so that we may still avail ourselves of its potent therapeutic activity.

This fear of toxic drugs was born at the beginning of the last century, after physicians had indulged for some time in an orgy of polypharmacy recalling those Persian physicians of Avicenna's time, who stuffed countless medicines from bottles as colorful as peacock plumes down the throats of the sick in the streets of Baghdad and Samarkand. The psychologic reaction to such medical bacchanalia was a deep fear of toxic drugs.

The investigation of antibiotics has reminded the physician of one of those truths so elemental that they are often forgotten, namely, that in pharmacology, with some notable exceptions, the most toxic agents are also the most active. Many antibiotics would never have been used clinically had their discoverers been prematurely frightened by their toxicity. Instead, aware of the fact that sometimes the greater the toxicity the more active the antibiotic, they proceeded to study how to reduce such toxicity. In theory, the most potent antibiotic would be the one that destroys the protoplasm not only of the bacterial cell but also of the human cell that houses it. This is equivalent to putting out a fire by destroying the burning house. In practice, however, we try to extinguish the fire and save both the house and its occupants.

A NEW RESPECT FOR MICROBES

Antibiotics have acquainted many physicians, who never dreamed that one day they would dabble in microbiology, with a series of fascinating facts about bacterial life and have aroused an increasing philosophic interest in the world of microbes. The modern physician, aware that our planet is made smaller each day by the airplane, to paraphrase Chesterton, compensates for this contraction of his universe by making it larger through the microscope.

Bacterial resistance to drugs is making the physician realize that as soon as a disease appears to be under control new problems arise.

Twenty years ago it was believed that gonorrhea could be controlled with sulfonamides, but it was soon discovered that certain cases resisted them. The same thing is now happening with infections that resist antibiotics. The physician is beginning to understand that in his struggle against infection two factors are involved: his own science, aided by chemotherapeutic resources, and the microbe itself; between the two a fascinating game of chess is being played in which the human body is the chessboard and the life of the patient is the prize. As in a ballet *pas de deux,* it is necessary for each participant to anticipate the reactions of the other if the dance is to reach a successful end. The microbe defends itself by resisting the drugs and developing new forms of attack. Hence the aphorism: "Be quick to use a remedy while it is still effective."

Research in antibiotics is therefore intimately connected with the progress of studies in microbiology and chemistry.* This fact has contributed to the forging of a new and solid bond between the physician and the laboratory scientist, so long separated, and to the creation of two new types of specialists—the clinical pharmacologist and the laboratory pathologist.†

------

* As S. Mudd has said about bacteria: "The structure revealed up to now by the electronic microscope is much more simple than that apparently required by the outstanding synthetic aptitudes of microorganisms. The bacterial cell, by receiving only water, salts, glucose, and simple supplies of carbon and nitrogen, is able to synthesize proteins, complex carbohydrates, lipids, ribose, nucleic acid, growth factors and enzymes, all of them organized in a characteristic and reproducible protoplasmic system. The bacterial cell can reproduce itself in half an hour at the temperature of the human body. This feat of chemical synthesis and organization, which could not be duplicated by the best chemical laboratory, is accomplished within a cell a few microns long and less than a micron in diameter. These simple facts would be fantastic were they not already familiar to us." (*Nature,* London. *161*:312.)

This teaches us a lesson in humility by reminding us that there are still many things that we do not know, things existing not in some galaxy of the universe millions of light-years away, not at the bottom of some abysmal ocean, but right in front of us and even within ourselves.

† Let us not forget that the production of a new chemotherapeutic agent by an organic chemist is the result of a prolonged pharmacologic investigation, based on knowledge derived from experimental work in pure physiology. New progress in chemotherapy depends on the progress of organic chemistry. Biochemistry is also making many contributions to chemotherapy and pharmacology. Sir Henry Dale's idea of the specific inhibition of biologic reactions was first developed and illustrated by Quastel and his associates, who studied the biochemical properties of the simple enzyme systems. Applied by Woods and Fildes to the metabolic processes of microorganisms, that concept formed the basis of an accepted theory of the activity of chemotherapies. This biochemical discovery will be one of the most important bases for future progress in chemotherapy and in many other branches of medical research.

But antibiotic medicine had to encounter, as a matter of course, the same grave danger faced by every new remedy in every epoch of history: the possible return to the psychologic beginnings of medical magic.

When the word "magic" is used, we physicians smile patronizingly, for we know that our convictions are based on the Gibraltar of scientific knowledge behind whose ramparts we are securely entrenched. Yet, we must remember that the towering castle of modern scientific medicine is built over the dark caves of primitive medical magic. We must remember that just as a civilized man may, in a moment of panic, revert to his deepest psychologic stratum—that hypothalamic entrenchment wherein our first prehistoric ancestor, with claws, fangs and all, still dwells—so even the most scientific physician may unconsciously return to a "scientific" magic, a magic as dangerous as that of the primitive medicine man.

Magic medicine was concerned only with the *who,* the *where,* and the *when:* the man who healed, the place where he healed, and the time when he healed. (The witch doctor performed his healing ceremonies in a magic cave and usually at midnight.) Scientific medicine is concerned only with the *what* and the *how:* what medicine to use and how it acts.

One recent manifestation of "scientific" magic was the belief in the omnipotence of certain antibiotics, which later proved to be completely disillusioning to both physician and patient. There are still many people to whom an ampule of penicillin or any other antibiotic —the newer the better—holds the same magic promise that a talisman or religious image held in times past. This has engendered the dangerous practice of self-medication, with the unfortunate secondary reactions consequent to the blind use of the so-called miracle drugs.

The "scientific" magic to which I refer stems from a certain intoxication that overcomes the physician of today when he feels that, with the aid of chemistry, bacteriology, physics, radiology, and mathematics, medicine is at last becoming an exact science; when he notes the effect of disease on humors and tissues, compares it with the similar effect of the medication, and reduces the whole to an algebraic equation, to a mathematical formula wherein everything is contained except the diseased person as an integral personality. Not in vain has it been said that it becomes easier every day to be a physician and more difficult to be a patient.

But the world's great clinicians, reacting logically, are struggling to reintegrate the findings of the laboratory, medical statistics, naturalistic clinical observation, and all pertinent scientific data into a wholesome Hippocratic criterion, without which no drug or contrivance can cure the patient. Or, even if he were physically cured, he might be left with a battered soul.

THE MAGIC OF THE THREE DOSES

An example of the survival of magic in the medical routine of today is the ritual of giving drugs three or four times a day. This ritual, as a Swedish psychiatrist, Ada Glynn, commented recently, has been handed down to us from the time of primitive medical magic. For the medical historian, this custom of giving drugs three or four times daily is associated with the primitive belief in the power of certain mystic numbers. The ancient Egyptians believed in a four-day cure. On the island of Eddystone every form of therapy lasts four days and sometimes it is repeated for four days every month for four consecutive months.

If we were to study pharmacologically the advisability of giving certain drugs three or four times a day and took into consideration the duration of the effect of each dose, we would see with surprise that in many cases there would be an overdosage and in others an underdosage, entailing in either case a great risk. Just the same, physicians continue to follow the practice of the three daily doses.

Although the administration of a drug is maintained within a certain margin of therapeutic dosage, patients with totally different constitutions are given exactly the same dose. If the desired effect is not achieved with one drug, another drug is tried, when actually what should be done is to determine the correct dosage required by the patient before—in cases of poor toleration—discarding a drug. The magical formula of *t.i.d.*, regardless of the patient's capacity to absorb or excrete the drug, sometimes makes the patient tolerant to drugs administered at short intervals.

We should be grateful for the new philosophy of dosage introduced by the antibiotics. Based on a careful determination of the duration of the effect of these drugs, their hematic and tissular levels, and the patient's reactions to them, this new philosophy is destroying numerical magic and replacing it with dosage schedules based on the solid reality of laboratory tests, mirrors that clearly reflect the effectiveness of a drug within the body of the patient.

THE IMPACT OF ANTIBIOTICS ON SURGERY AND
ON MEDICAL SPECIALTIES

The practicing physician is a witness to the drastic change that the face of modern medicine is undergoing. Antibiotics have forced surgery to retreat to second place and to adopt a conservative attitude, in sharp contrast with the historically aggressive attitude of those surgeons who, armed with their glittering scalpels, took possession of medicine at the beginning of this century. Antibiotics have also caused a decrease in medical specialties. The number of patients being rescued from surgery by antibiotic medicine (only the dramatic abdominal and cerebral surgery is still in the forefront of the medical picture) is increasing every day; successful treatment with antibiotics of many infectious processes of the urinary tract, which formerly required years of painful and inefficient treatment, and of ear, nose, and throat infections have made urology and otorhinolaryngology fade away as "semisurgical" specialties before the antibiotic offensive.

These indisputable facts imply the philosophic theory that modern medicine is becoming more concerned with eternal than with immediate matters. Surgery is, above all, action and urgency, a struggle against the clock, the rebellion of the surgeon's hands against the tyranny of time. Antibiotic medicine, because it is based on scientific research which represents eternity, attacks disease quietly and from solid biologic strongholds rather than with the "commando" tactics of surgery.

In the best of cases, the physician of yesterday was a *minister Naturae,* a servant of nature who helped along the natural processes of healing. The physician who today uses antibiotics is no longer a servant but a master of nature, *magister Naturae,* for he tries to control disease by guiding with his knowledge the natural processes themselves. The modern physician therefore combines two different roles—*magister* and *minister* of nature—when he accomplishes by means of antibiotics a work of art that nature herself could not imitate.

Frequently, when there is no other way, the physician calls to his aid legions of microbes, which he pits against other microbes in an invisible civil war even more ferocious than atomic warfare. The physician who uses certain microbes as his allies against the microbes that are his adversaries is repeating the invocation of Juno in Vergil's *Aeneid: "Flectere, si nequeo Superos Acheronta movebo."* ("If the Gods do not come to my aid, I shall call upon legions of demons.")

A CHANGE IN THE DISEASES OF THE FUTURE

The profound change that is taking place in the natural history of infections warrants the prophecy that by the year 2000 the diseases caused by bacteria, protozoa, and perhaps viruses will be considered by the medical student as exotic curiosities of mere historical interest, as is the case today with tertiary syphilis, gout, and smallpox. On the other hand, as "old" diseases disappear, "new" ones spring up, as was the case in 1918 with epidemic encephalitis, and recently with the hemorrhagic fevers registered in Korea. Cases of neurodystrophy, cancer, arteriosclerosis, and psychosis will probably increase. Diseases that formerly were deadly, such as pneumonia, which Osler once called "captain of the men of death," can today be treated more successfully than a simple cold, but "new" diseases now baffle medical science. For man's greatest danger lies precisely in his being human.

Antibiotics therefore are changing the face of humanity, replacing the juvenile face it wore in the times of classical Greece, when men lived a short time and died young, with the white-haired, wrinkled face characteristic of longevity. For as a result of the almost radical elimination of the infections that formerly decimated the world's population, man's lifespan has greatly increased, with the consequent increase in the proportion of old people.*

True, pneumonia, typhoid, and other infections are being replaced by leukemia, cardiopathy, psychosis, and cancer; but even so, with the disappearance of the infections that used to cause 25 per cent of all deaths, the population of the planet is becoming a population of old people with all the sociologic consequences implied therein.†

We do not yet know the effect that antibiotics will have on the human organism. I am an optimist; I do not join in the pessimistic prophecies that maintain that the use of antibiotics will eventually have fearsome effects. Hormones can be noxious if they are abused, and cases of premature aging caused by the misuse of vitamins have likewise been reported. The use of antibiotics, as of all potent medications, requires a continuous study in the laboratory and experimentation not only on animals but also on human beings.

THE DUTY TO EXPERIMENT CLINICALLY

Clinical experimentation on human beings is imperative in the field of antibiotics. There are human diseases that cannot be exactly reproduced in laboratory animals. One kilogram of body weight of a rat or rabbit cannot be equated *mutatis mutandis* with one kilogram of human body weight. As the Spanish medical philosopher Letamendi said: "In human medicine there are too few men and too many frogs." (*"En la Medicina humana, falta hombre y sobra rana."*)

----

* It is an interesting observation that most antibiotics were discovered by men fully mature or in a still creative old age. It is as if, grateful for having reached the biologic sunset of life still in possession of full mental powers, they wished to make a precious offering to those men who died young from infections that are successfully treated today.

† In the time of Sydenham, "fevers" represented seventy-five per cent of all medical cases; today, if we exclude influenza epidemics, they represent only five per cent.

The founder of experimental medicine, Claude Bernard, once said: *"Pour savoir quelque chose sur les fonctions de la vie il faut les étudier sur le vivant."* ("To learn something about the functions of life one must study them in the living.") *"Tout médecin savant doit donc avoir un laboratoire physiologique."* Today the clinic has become this physiologic laboratory which, according to Claude Bernard, every physician should have. In this thought the great philosopher anticipated the portentous progress made in clinical pharmacology and the countless tests of new drugs made on hospital patients, which offer a ray of hope to millions of human beings throughout the world.

THE WORK OF THE PHARMACEUTICAL INDUSTRY: CHAIRS OF ANTIBIOTIC MEDICINE

What we have said applies not only to the practice of medicine and antibiotic science but also to medical instruments. *"La médecine expérimentale doit sa solidité, son honnêteté, aux appareils,"* said Charles Niccole. If experimental medicine owes its solidity and honesty to medical instruments, then the physician must call upon those who can supply them. We must again listen to Claude Bernard: *"Souvent même certaines questions scientifiques exigent impérieusement pour pouvoir être résolues des instruments coûteux et compliqués de sorte qu'on peut dire alors que la question scientifique est véritablement subordonnée à une question d'argent."* ("Often the solutions of certain scientific problems imperiously demand costly and complicated instruments; it can be said that the problem of science is truly subordinated to the problem of money.")

This makes it fitting that we should all thank the pharmaceutical industry for its vast and valuable contribution. We may say that they have hastened the pace of history itself; by struggling against time, they have caused research in antibiotics to don the legendary seven-league boots and stride bravely forward.

The day that the pharmaceutical companies, which have already done so much to spread medical culture in the field of antibiotics, understand the necessity of systematizing this culture, of giving it an organic form, and of building it with a perspective toward eternity— that day they will establish throughout the world the Chairs of Antibiotic Medicine that I have already proposed. I again propose these Chairs, not only as an ideal but as an additional duty, the fulfillment of which can cover the pharmaceutical industry with glory, since they would be bequeathing an invaluable educational service to the medical generations of the future.

THE PHYSICIAN ABOVE THE DRUGS

Until now we have spoken about the importance of antibiotics in the professional and scientific life of the modern physician. I wish to devote a few words to the importance of the physician as a professional and as a man concerned with the progress of antibiotic medicine.

There is something even more marvelous than the technical discoveries that light the picture of modern medicine or the instruments and drugs in use today: I refer, of course, to the man behind them, the man whose knowledge can restore the sick to health—the physician.

What really cures a sick person—and let us not forget this lest we fall back again into the dangers of magic medicine—is not merely the use of drugs or instruments, for the instruments cannot make a diagnosis by themselves, nor can drugs alone effect a cure. The cure is achieved by the man who knows how to use these drugs and instruments correctly and effectively. An antibiotic no more cures an infection than a scalpel cures peritonitis. It is the brains and the hands of the physician or surgeon that perform the miracle of healing. The marvelous resources at our disposal would be of no great avail if they were not used by men skilled in their profession.

The relationship between a patient and a physician is not a generic relationship between an infection and an antibiotic: it is a specific relationship between two human beings, one sick and suffering and the other endowed with the knowledge necessary to treat him. The final cure is accomplished by a combination of factors involving the nature of the patient, the characteristics of his infection, the knowledge of the physician, and the curative resources at his disposal. Under the guidance of the physician, antibiotics perform their curative miracle. And if the practicing physician should pay tribute to the laboratory research worker, whose achievements make possible the progress of scientific medicine, the latter should also render homage to the clinical practitioner who, possessing the "science and conscience" that Montaigne spoke of, accomplishes the final cure.

To believe. To reason. To experiment. Faith, philosophy, and science will always be the trilogy that inspires the physician and the research worker. Because both physician and research scientist are looking for God in their own fashion, whether by the flickering light of a candle at the bedside of a sick farmer or by the bright light, so reminiscent of twinkling stars, of the Bunsen burners in a laboratory.

THE DUTY TO SPEAK AND WRITE

I would like my final words to be a summons to the practicing physician to widen the horizon of his scientific culture in antibiotics every day, and to the research worker to become more and more acquainted with clinical medicine. And both should constantly keep in mind their duty to communicate through medical journals what they observe, deduce, discover, or prove.

The physician today has a special obligation: to speak and write about what he sees and knows, and to do so as clearly, harmoniously, and euphonically as he can.

In Greek mythology, as W. R. Betts once observed, the favorite son of Apollo, god of beauty, culture, rhetoric, poetry, and light, was Aesculapius, on whom the gods conferred the divine gift of healing. Ever since, faithful to the memory of the friendship that once existed between poetry and "physic," physicians have called themselves children of Apollo. In the Renaissance, medicine was part of every student's education, just as literature was part of every physician's curriculum. In contrast with those times of avid curiosity and desire to learn everything, many modern physicians prefer to live shut up in a single room of the vast palace of medicine instead of exploring the rest of the castle. The time has come for physicians to realize that medical work, whether clinical or investigative, should be done with the joy—*cito, tute et jucunde*—that characterized the physicians of classical Greece and illuminated the pages of William Osler and Oliver Wendell Holmes.

Let us then, children of Apollo, try to maintain a harmonious balance between our work and our dreams, our serious endeavors and our joy in living, so that we, as physicians, may keep our appointment with glory and, as men, our rendezvous with life.

THE NEXT HALF CENTURY IN ANTIBIOTIC MEDICINE AND ITS EFFECT ON THE HISTORY OF THE CLINICAL CASE HISTORY

THE BEST HISTORICAL DOCUMENT

*W*hen we wish to know the secret of a man's or a nation's greatness, we usually look up its "official" history; but just as a single drop of water can yield all the elements of the sea, so can a mere glimpse at a sketch collecting dust on a shelf in a great artist's studio yield the clue to his innermost yearnings and so to the secret of his fame; or so can a random glance through an open window at the blazing hearth of a contented family yield the key to a nation's greatness.

If I were asked what sort of documents I would choose to comprehend better the medical history of any one period, I would choose not the biographies of the great scientists, not even an enumeration of the great medical discoveries in that period; I would choose a representative clinical case history scribbled by a physician at the bedside of his patient. For such a humble document indeed affords a live, meaningful summary of the clinical know-how of an age, archetypically represented in the practical wisdom of a general practitioner. No other document can throw as much light on the evolution of medical knowledge through the centuries as the ordinary clinical case history.

The history of medicine is generally written with an eye only for medical giants, great discoveries, and famous institutions. But all this is only façade and contingency. The basic facts, the true meaning of

Delivered at the Third Annual Symposium on Antibiotics, Washington, D. C., November 2–4, 1955.

the history of medicine, all are contained in the humble clinical case history—that "small change" of medicine—written by an anonymous practitioner in an office or in a hospital.

No more authentic history of the evolution of medical thought could be written than by compiling and analyzing clinical case histories from Hippocrates down to our time.

Using the clinical case history as a backdrop, we shall attempt here to project into the future what we think may happen in the next half century in antibiotic medicine.

We especially chose antibiotic medicine because often certain medical discoveries determine the character of the medicine of the next century. This is what happened with the work of Vesalius, Harvey, and Pasteur. It also happened with Fleming and his followers, who made of the twentieth century the Antibiotic Age. Let us see what we can learn about the next half century of this Antibiotic Age by studying the changes wrought by antibiotics in the history of the clinical case history. But first we must define what we mean by *clinical case history*.

WHAT IS A CLINICAL CASE HISTORY?

A clinical case history is the record of the physician's historical attitude when facing the problem of disease and the living reality of the patient.

The history of medicine is not the chronologic story of the evolution of the men, ideas, and places that participated in the construction of that complex scaffolding we call present-day medical science. It is rather—and here we agree with Spengler's and Toynbee's ideas on the meaning of history—the story of a series of historic situations, strung together in the course of time, in each of which the physician tried to cure the patient by recalling age-old wisdom, by utilizing his own experience, and by exercising his intuition as to what might happen in the future.

The clinical case history records the physician's attempts to assist the patient in each of those historic situations. The history of the clinical case history is therefore the most authentic, and consequently the most scientific, of all the many possible approaches to the history of medicine.

ON THE HISTORY OF THE CLINICAL CASE HISTORY

The clinical case history was actually born with the forty-two pathographic accounts written by Hippocrates in the first and third books of his *Epidemics*. Before Hippocrates we find summary sketches of clinical pictures on old Egyptian papyri; but only in the work of the Father of Medicine do we find the first clinical histories or *cathastases,* a term that covers not only a highly individualized account of what happens to a patient, but also a description of his environment and of the nosologic entity that affects him. Hippocratic *cathastases* were compiled for the purpose of leaving, as a guide for future physicians, a record of diseases actually observed in patients.

After several centuries of sterile Byzantine and Arabic groping, the Hippocratic *cathastases* were followed by medieval *consilia,* like those of Arnold of Villanova, which were as universal in scope as the Hippocratic accounts were individualized; they were concerned with disease as an abstract entity rather than with the individual patient, and their objective was, as its name suggests, to counsel the physician. The naturalistic intention therefore gave way to the didactic motive. The Hippocratic *cathastase* was a naturalistic account; the medieval *consilium* was a didactic dissertation.

The medieval *consilia* lasted from the thirteenth to the sixteenth centuries, when, with the advent of the Renaissance *observationes,* a new concept of the clinical history was born. Individualization and humanization of the clinical report prevailed again, and new, mainly anatomic, elements appeared, relating disease to the lesions it causes, this being a reflection of the impact of Vesalius.

The Renaissance *observationes* were gradually integrated into the *historiae morbi* of the seventeenth century, after which Thomas Sydenham introduced a new pathographic concept of the clinical history which made of the patient a jumping-off point for the description of diseases: "disease species" as classifiable as a naturalist's butterflies or a paleontologist's bones. Thus the patient became the loom on which Sydenham's clinical history wove a multicolored tapestry of diseases.

From the seventeenth to the nineteenth centuries, first by Boerhaave and finally by Bichat, the anatomicoclinical concept of the clinical history was elaborated. The patient was no longer isolated on his island of pain, but rather the anatomicoclinical basis of his disease was emphasized. This type of clinical history was later joined to physiopathologic accounts, especially those by neurologists like J. Hughlings Jackson who correlated symptoms, signs, anatomic lesions, and physiopathologic disturbances.

When Laënnec introduced the stethoscope, the clinical case history, which had been visual for almost two thousand years, became auditive. Three new auditive factors took on sudden importance in the clinical case history, which until then had been the product of sight and pen: the pathologic sound (murmurs, stertors); the patient's groans; and the patient's words, in anamnesis, more and more carefully recorded.

Later, at the end of the last century, two new factors came into play: the *etiopathogenic component,* which had gained in importance since Pasteur introduced the microbial doctrine of infection and caused the clinical picture to have meaning only in terms of the causal microbe or the etiopathogenic element; and the *pathobiographic and anthropologic approach* of Freud, who introduced the personal biography into the clinical case history and endowed the auditive factor with sudden importance as the patient's complexes, invisible to the eye, began to "be heard." Disease, then, was considered—as von Weizsäcker and the psychosomatic school showed—not as an accident or unhealthy deviation in the patient's life, but as an integral, active part of that life, as a basic *way of life.*

FEATURES OF THE CURRENT CLINICAL CASE HISTORY

The clinical case history today is the result of the confluence of these historical currents and is characterized by several factors: (1) it is not written, as it once was, by a single physician, but is the result of the collaboration of a team of specialists whose opinions are integrated by the attending physician; (2) it attaches great importance to laboratory reports[A] and, in so doing, breaks the patient down into facts and figures that reveal the state of his blood, urine, lungs, and metabolic chemistry; (3) it attaches a limited importance—except in psychiatric clinical case histories—to the patient's "total person," to the real essence of the living being; (4) it still forgets to a great extent the biographic account and stresses the accident of infection more than the concurrence of factors that placed the patient at that intersection of a moment of time and a fragment of space where the infection took place; (5) it stresses the therapeutic element, almost forgotten in Hippocratic clinical case histories and eliminated altogether during the period of therapeutic nihilism, thus making therapy the basic factor in the clinical case history not only as a curative element, but as a diagnostic aid when the patient's reactions to therapy are evaluated; (6) it introduces the environmental factor, made all-important by the present-day social structure, for now the patient's prognosis includes information, that may help his family, his employers, and the society in which he lives to determine when and in what conditions he may again participate in the activities from which disease temporarily isolated him; (7) it attaches special importance to the educational and medical communication factors, for it includes the observations made on the use of diagnostic techniques on the patient, as well as the effects of accepted therapeutic methods, all for the enlightenment of future physicians.

If we examine the clinical history of infections at the various stages in the history of medicine, we see that each one of its component factors has successively governed these stages and has thus governed the cultural panorama of the medicine of each age.

Thus, during Hippocrates' time the *whole* patient dominated the clinical case history and was the chief preoccupation of the practicing physician; from Galen to Sydenham, the philosophic notion of the disease as a nosologic entity prevailed; from Pasteur to Fleming, the etiologic agent became the hero of the clinical case history, which concentrated more on recounting the details of bacteriologic investigation into the causal germ than on the effect the microbe had on the patient. Since the introduction of antibiotics, therapy is the axis around which revolves the clinical case history and, therefore, the entire picture of contemporary medicine.

Today the clinical case history of an infectious patient attaches more importance to the therapeutic measures adopted—not always wisely or successfully—than to investigation of the picture of the disease and the patient's reaction to microbial aggression.

THE INTEGRATING FACTORS OF THE CLINICAL CASE HISTORY,
TODAY AND TOMORROW

The elements therefore constituting today the clinical case history of an infectious patient are the following: (1) *the patient,* considered as a field of study and action for the physician; (2) *the disease,* as a nosologic entity; (3) *the microbe,* as an etiopathogenic factor; (4) *the anti-infectious* therapy, as an expression of the physician's fight against the disease, represented mainly by antibiotics; (5) *the environment* of the patient, whence he came and where he will return once he is cured, represented by his family and society; (6) *the educational* aspects of the clinical case history, which make it an important means of medical communication.

Let us now look at each one of these factors and point out briefly how we consider them today and, projected by our present knowledge, how they may be considered in the next half century, as the Ship of Time sails toward the year 2000.

THE SIX ELEMENTS OF A CLINICAL CASE HISTORY

I. The patient as a "case" and as a sick person.

The patient, including the infectious patient, appears in today's clinical case history in a light quite different from a half century ago.

Before the formulation of the microbial theory, the patient was a "thing" that could be understood by studying its physical symptoms. But since Klebs, the patient has been looked upon as the battlefield for the biologic war waged between his organism and the infecting germs. From being a "thing" the patient became a living being, capable of responding to the cause of disease in a way that guaranteed his survival. The patient's body ceased to be a mere theatre housing the drama of disease, and became an organism in a dramatic biologic action. Thus, three supreme attributes of the sick person were accepted: his *totality,* that is, his humoral and psychoneuroendocrine unity; his individual *constitution,* which conditions the response to the microbial aggression in disease; and his *responsiveness,* which makes each symptom a response to the new situation created by the disease.

The physician at the end of the last century was pre-eminently the classic "family doctor": he knew and understood his patients and their environment thoroughly. But during the intermezzo between the two world wars (1918–1939), the physician, intoxicated by the new technical tools, relied more on diagnostic elements, on x-rays and the laboratory, than on his own senses, on auscultation and percussion. In this manner the flesh and blood patient was forgotten; instead there was created that medical abstraction called "the clinical case," e.g., "the diabetic," "the typhoidic," "the addisonian."

Thus, in interpreting the phenomenon of disease, the same error was committed as is often made by tourists visiting a cave of stalactites and stalagmites: A guide may point out that the fantastic formations resemble palaces, crypts, phallic symbols, and soon the tourists can see nothing else but the symbols evoked by the imagination. Similarly, when many physicians of half a century ago interpreted the phenomenon of infection, they saw only germs, just as some physicians today see only psychosomatic reactions. In reality, in order to understand the phenomenon of disease, we must take into account not only the germ and the body that harbors it, but also the interaction between both that produces the disease.

But the tendency still followed today by many physicians is to extend the horizon of the etiologic concern that started with Pasteur at the end of the last century, continued with Koch and Lister, and was developed by Ehrlich and Domagk. They still focus the treatment of a disease on its etiology as a means of erasing with one fell swoop the vast mural of symptoms and signs of clinical pathology. They forget that, besides the "etiologic sign" which still plays top role in physicians' minds, they should also look for the sick person who exists behind the infection.

The clinician's objective today, which will certainly throw light on the concept of the patient in the next half century, is, in all cases of infection, not only to destroy the microbe and eradicate the infection but to bring about *cito, tuto et jocunde,* quickly, completely, and felicitously, the recovery of the patient.

It is imperative therefore that we revise the prevalent philosophic notion of the treatment of infections, and reconcile the nosologic and the etiopathogenic concepts of disease. As the pendulum of history swings back to its point of origin, there is a revival of the neo-Hippocratic concept: that of treating the *whole* patient, as we do today, for example, when we combine antibiotics with vitamins in anti-infectious therapies.

Until about ten years ago, infection was considered the result of a pathogenic microorganism lodged in the propitious soil that was the patient's organism. However, with the development of specific anti-infectious chemotherapy, the feeling was that the problem of infection could be solved in the same way that a chess problem is solved: if the therapeutic chessmen were played in a certain way, the infection would be mathematically checkmated.

The Hippocratic notion of taking care of the patient and treating the infected area was replaced by a mathematical notion. Each microbe was considered as flying game for the hunter; the physician aimed his therapeutic gun at it and fired the magic bullets of a specific chemotherapy. But one thing was forgotten—the *sick* human being harboring the infection.

When Selye introduced the concept of stress, with infection as one of its causes—not in terms of the specific organic response to the microbial agent, but of the capacity of the germ to cause a nonspecific stress—he revived interest not only in treating the infection from the etiologic point of view, but also in safeguarding the total nutritional personality of the patient.

In the clinical case history of the next half century we shall probably attach due importance to the whole person of the infectious patient, and we shall not allow the growing specificity of the therapy to lessen the nonspecificity of the patient's hygiene, without which no etiologic therapy can have satisfactory results.

Although chemotherapy may completely destroy the etiologic agent of an infection, the patient—consumed by the stress caused by disease, with its vitamin depletion and shortage of proteins and mineral salts—may also very well be destroyed; for it must never be forgotten that besides the microbe that must be destroyed, there is a patient who must be cured.

The clinical case history of the infectious patient in the next half century will therefore be more "biographic" and less purely therapeutic, and therefore will reflect not only a great deal of laboratory data but also the *whole* image of the patient.

II. The new concept of disease, including infection.

The second aspect of the clinical case history that may change radically in the next half century is the philosophic concept of the nature of disease, which is already undergoing a revolutionary transition.

The primitive medicine man was not interested in the nature of disease, but only in its cure, and he availed himself of various doctrines—similarity, analogy and contagion—to explain its genesis.

From the beginning of history there have been two antagonistic concepts of disease: the *ontologic,* which derives from the belief that a diseased person is possessed by a demon and which considers disease as an autonomous entity taking a regular course and endowed with a natural history; and the *biographic* or *historical,* which records disease as one more event in the individual life of the patient.[B]

To the ontologic concept belong Glisson's and Sydenham's clinical descriptions, plus present-day descriptions of clinical pictures of typhoid, epilepsy, and other diseases made by certain physicians who still think that the pathognomonic signs are valuable diagnostic short cuts, unaware as they are that, from the point of view of a later therapy, such a diagnosis is insufficient.

Today we accept the clinical labels of disease, including infections, as convenient symbols for describing clinical pictures that are often isomorphic, like acromegaly or Parkinson's disease; but these labels are unsatisfactory when the clinical picture is variable, as occurs in the case of rheumatoid arthritis or schizophrenia. Among the dangers implicit in this concept of diseases as *disease entities* figures the mechanization of the physician.

In contradiction to this tendency there is a growing concept of disease as a *deviation from normality;* in this way we establish *anatomic* syndromes (like those caused by an imbalance in carbohydrate tolerance) and *pathologic* syndromes (like those caused by inflammation or congenital syphilis).

This concept of disease accepts the fact that its signs and symptoms, often reproduced in constant patterns, indicate one or more of three aspects of the disease: its *location,* the *associated functional disturbances,* and its *causal factors* expressed in terms of pathology, physiology, psychology, and ecology.[C] The next half century will see the rise of this new concept of the nature of disease.

In the new concepts, the relationship between cause and effect in organic diseases has already changed. Instead of "specific causes," we speak of interrelationships and correlations between the seed and the terrain, and of series of pathologic events linked in the body of the patient.

More and more, diseases, including infections, are considered as intersections in time and space of what has been called "time-sequence." An infection, therefore, turns out to be the "germ-time sequence crossing the patient-time sequence."

MEN, MOLDS, AND HISTORY

More and more each year we seek out concomitant causes instead of merely searching for the main etiologic factor. Modern psychiatry furnished medicine with a valuable research tool when it showed how to establish a multidimensional etiologic diagnosis. In the next half century this technique will also be applied to the pathology of infection.

In infectious cases, the physician in the next fifty years will no longer be concerned, as his predecessor was at the beginning of the century, mainly with the fact that pneumococcus always produces pneumonia—which is not really true since pneumococcus may, depending on its location, produce a meningitis as well as a pneumonia —but rather with the basic factors of infection, i.e., the patient, the environment, and the mechanism of interaction between the two. He will therefore determine *how* the patient lived, *why* he became sick (study of the environment), and *what* his illness is, considered as a series of mechanisms of interaction.

We have come to the conclusion that disease cannot exist outside the human body, whether it be in books, jars of alcohol, morgues, or laboratories. All disease, whether it be rickets or schizophrenia, requires an organic structure in which to develop.

In the next half century it will be generally accepted that man is the result of three factors: his genetic origin, his environment, and his free will. Disease will be considered the process of a human being showing, at a given moment in his life, structural or functional alterations, complicated by the effect of psychosomatic interactions between his genetic and constitutional factors and his adverse environmental factors.

The psychiatrist von Weizsäcker has suggested dividing diseases into three groups, on which the clinical diagnoses of the next half century may perhaps be based: (a) *neuroses,* or atemporal functional alterations in the rhythm, direction and proportion of the phenomena of absorption, secretion, chemism, and movement, endowed with social repercussions; (b) *bioses,* or reversible and transient alterations of the cellular structures, infections, neoformations, and degenerations of a more inert course and manifest in the whole body of the individual; and (c) *scleroses,* or irreversible structural alterations representing the "historical" aspect of disease and located in one part of the body.

The physician's objective in the next half century will be to translate into practical reality this new concept of disease, dealing with disease—neuroses, bioses, and scleroses—from a triple point of view: improving the human being eugenically; improving his environment by means of hygienic measures applied to individual and collective life; and changing the psychosomatic constitution of the human being medically through physical, biochemotherapeutic, and psychologic methods in order to improve his way of reacting to disease.

In the next half century, diseases, including infections, will be accepted by the physician as a painful, anomalous way of life that he must wholly understand if he is to correct.

III. The biologic value of germs and their modification by means of antibiotics.

And now let us discuss another vital component of the clinical case history of the infectious patient: the germs—and what they will mean to the physician in the next half century.

The next half century will confirm that it is important to learn to live with the germs around us and to accept the limitations that such association imposes on the use of antibiotics. Not all microbes are man's implacable enemies. Without microbes all life would soon disappear from the face of the earth.

All animals depend on vegetable life for their food, whether they subsist on plants only or on other herbivorous animals. If all bacteria disappeared, the nitrogen cycle of the soil would be interrupted and plants would stop growing. And so there would be temporarily an aseptic humanity, but soon because of lack of food all life would come to an end.

If the physician did not regard disease only from an anthropocentric point of view, he would understand that infection is not something accidental, but rather the logical consequence of the interactions between the different forms of life on earth. All forms of earth life maintain among them an unstable equilibrium. An epidemic simply represents the temporary triumph of causal germs when they upset this balance.

Microbial resistance to the new drugs, plus the fact that if we destroy too many pathogenic bacteria the viruses, taking advantage of the imbalance thus caused in nature, will increase and unleash epidemics, would prove Pasteur's dream of a world free of all germs to be utopian.

It may be that, since the beginning of the Chemotherapeutic Era and the elimination of germs susceptible to antibiotics, the world is gradually becoming populated with new breeds of bacteria as virulent as those that have disappeared, and which are safe from us, at least until we discover a new antibiotic to destroy them.

Just as the world would be in grave danger if insectivorous animals disappeared and carnivorous animals were free to develop to gigantic proportions, so would the healthy man be in grave danger if we tampered with the balance in his body of certain germs indispensable to his survival and health.

A bacteriologically aseptic and parasitologically pure man, if such a human being could exist at all, would suffer serious growth and nutritional disturbances and would be the victim of severe infections such as could not be conceived by modern pathology. Antibiotic therapy, if indiscriminately used, may turn out to be a medicinal flood that temporarily cleans and heals, but ultimately destroys life itself by carrying off germs indispensable to that very life.

Just as thieves and criminals force communities to maintain a vigilant police force, so parasitism forces the organism to keep its own defenses in a state of constant vigilance. Were it not for the alarm caused by such germs, the body's natural defenses would be lulled to sleep or perhaps would not even exist, and at the first infection man would succumb.

Is this then to be the "revenge" of the germs against the antibiotics? For ultimately they will unquestionably benefit by the destruction of the host's cellular resistance, and this destruction is possible, as the organism, depending more and more on antibiotics for protection, may become "lazy" and cease to use those natural defensive humoral immunization mechanisms that it developed after millions of years of evolution and that until now constituted its most important means of defense.

The human organism must still fight its own battles; it must not be allowed to lapse into the habit of calling in a foreign army to fight in its stead. It is not possible to eliminate all dangerous germs or "microbe delinquency," because in every "raid" good germs are bound to be rounded up, thereby also weakening the organism's immunologic police force.

As germs increase in virulence, more powerful antibiotics will be discovered. In part at least, this medical progress is comparable to that of warfare: our bombs become more and more deadly, but so do the enemy's weapons. The best thing is to do without such weapons.

The next half century may witness a more conservative attitude toward the problem of microbes both within and outside man. Antibiotics that will attack pathogenic germs and respect saprophytics will be developed. We shall study in greater detail the natural history of every infection and the life cycle of each microbe in an endeavor to learn which are the weakest links in the biologic chain and attack them, respecting, however, the microbial balance in nature and in man. The physician may learn that the best way of overcoming enemy microbes is to respect their own biologic laws.

As part of this new more "respectful" approach to the microbial world, there may be born a new field of study: the combination of antibiotic therapy with enzymology and immunology, resulting in drugs that integrate antibiotics, enzymes, and biologicals. This will permit the physician to fight the pathogenic microbe and at the same time strengthen the humoral organic defenses of the human being.

And perhaps the greatest scientific accomplishment in store for mankind in the next half century may be the development of biochemical means that will enable man to live at peace or in "armed truce" with his enemies of the microbial world. The best way to overcome an enemy is to make of him a friend.

IV. Antibiotics in the next half century.

In figuring out what may happen to the antibiotics—the therapeutic component of the clinical case history—in the next half century, we must remember the change wrought in the clinical evaluation of medicines. Primitive man instinctively discovered many medicines, but he always used them along with magico-religious charms and incantations. Scientific medicine began the day drugs were prepared and administered independently of such magic rituals.

The principal anti-infectious therapy used today is antibiotics, which have, among other things, limited the field of surgical action. The knife has been exiled from certain parts of the body, thanks to the fulfillment of Ehrlich's prophetic statement: "The surgeon works with a steel scalpel; the chemotherapeutist with the chemical scalpel."

Antibiotics are constantly being accused of encouraging the development of bacteria-resistant strains, of causing superimposed infections activated by alterations in bacterial ecology, and of arousing secondary reactions. They also stand accused of changing the typical course of disease, thereby increasing diagnostic difficulties and creating new clinical pictures that will force physicians of the future to learn the picture of a disease after it has been modified by antibiotics.

We all deplore the abuses of this as well as of any other therapy. The ideal thing would be to use the "umbrella" of antibiotics only in real pathologic storms and not for passing summer showers. But the syndromes caused by antibiotics are only one more chapter in the picture of diseases caused by man. Such pathology will prevail as long as chemists continue to discover new compounds.

The critics of antibiotics should not forget that antibiotics have won a place for themselves, which they will never lose, in the anti-infectious arsenal.[D] Of course, antibiotics are at a disadvantage with respect to vaccines and serums, for they must wait for the disease to begin before being used clinically. Vaccines and serums have eradicated smallpox and tetanus in many areas, for they have swept the causal germs out of our environment or organism. Antibiotics will, in the future, "purify" many individuals who carry pathogenic streptococci, pneumococci, and other microbes, thus reducing the danger of contagion in daily life.

Antibiotics will protect the man of the future by destroying in his childhood those germs that might exist in his organism and environment, thus freeing him from many diseases of adulthood.

The next half century will probably reveal a double tendency in the field of antibiotic therapy: along with new broad-spectrum antibiotics capable of destroying almost any type of enemy bacteria, other antibiotics will be developed capable of reaching the most difficult target and having such specific and limited effect that they will destroy a *single* germ. We shall boast of chemical atom bombs and magic biochemical arrows.

That is why it is necessary to learn more and more about the enzymatic mechanisms of germs and develop antibiotics that will act as monkey wrenches in the microbial metabolic machinery, disorganizing and disrupting it, thereby facilitating the phagocytic sweeping out of germs.

Also, antibiotic therapy in the next half century will aim at more *prophylactic* and less therapeutic ends. It will become more preventive and less curative, for antibiotics will be used—for example, in pediatrics—mainly for prophylactic ends.

Let us not forget the symbolic example of Fleming, whose main interest in life was research into the natural defenses of the body—phagocytes, opsonins, and the body's own "antibiotic," lysozyme. For Fleming antibiotics were only a scientific interlude between the study of the infection and the study of immunity.

Research into new curative agents in the next half century will aim at integrating antibiotics with our natural organic defenses, thus combining artificial external attack with the natural internal defense against infection.

In our search for antibiotics we have examined samples of earth from all parts of the world. The next half century will witness similar explorations into the sea as a source of antibiotics, or we may investigate the antibiotics that exist in another natural source: the animal and human body.

V. Environment and the problem of the society of the future.

Now let us look briefly into the role that environment and society —important factors in the clinical case history—will play in the next half century.

Recently, the British scientist, Dr. George Thompson, outlined for us a world of the future in which monkeys, microbes, and machines will do man's work, allowing him more time for intellectual and artistic pursuits.

In such a society, monkeys would do the mechanical work today performed by men of low intellect; microbes would take care of all sorts of fermentation for industrial, medical, biologic, and nutritive uses; while machines, bolstered by all the advances made in cybernetics, would free us from the last of our present-day routines.

Even if we do not subscribe to such an optimistic outlook, we must agree that clinical pathology will be vastly different in the next half century. Hygiene and therapeutics will be more effective in their prophylactic aspects, and the average life span will exceed seventy-five years, consequently increasing geriatric and social problems.

Mortality in childhood and adolescence will decrease, thanks to social and preventive medicine, thus forcing people in good health to concern themselves with the discovery of latent diseases. The development of endocellular enzymology, key to biochemical mysteries, and initial therapy for incipient diseases—which is the same as saying prophylaxis in its final phases—will mean that fewer people will die young; consequently, more people will die of old age. This will create a growing concern with geriatric pathology, shocks and intoxications, vascular diseases, neuroses, and degenerative and psychiatric processes. And surgery will be limited to traumatology and congenital malformations.

Today's medical literature will be considered classic in the year 2000. The medical student of the end of this century will have to cope with a pathology devoted specially to neuroses, radioactive and industrial diseases, cancer, hardening of the arteries and degenerative diseases, and affections caused by stress and nonspecific agents, as contrasted with the highly specific infectious pathology of our time.

The microbes populating the air about us will probably follow two different courses: some germs, in waves of ever-decreasing virulence, will finally become saprophytes or will disappear altogether; others will develop new ways of resisting or overcoming the natural organic defenses.

We cannot, however, expect that because certain diseases are disappearing, causal germs will do the same. What has happened to those germs—for instance, diphtheria germs—that have apparently disappeared from our world? What happened to germs that were eliminated as a result of immunizations? These are biologic and chemical mysteries that the bacteriologist of the next half century will have to solve.

Because antibiotics are more effective in prolonging life than any other measure known, they will change the entire picture of our social structure and will force us to reorientate ourselves and our world in order to cope with new problems.

The situation will be the same as that facing a person who takes an express subway train instead of a local in order to save three minutes. What will he do with the three minutes he saved? Similarly we might ask ourselves: What will we do with the lives we have made longer and with the society of old people we are creating, thanks especially to antibiotics? The least we can do is to guarantee them that they will not perish from other causes and that they will have health. In turn, society will benefit from the experience, equanimity, wisdom, and good sense of the old people who will govern the world at the end of our century.

Fleming anticipated these problems when he said: "Cortisone and ACTH are playing their part in rheumatic diseases, and the introduction of chemotherapeutic drugs and more especially the antibiotics has diminished enormously death from many of our common infections. People are living longer and the population of the world is fast increasing. If the increased population is to remain healthy it must be well nourished. That means more food production. The doctors have done their work by increasing the expectations of life. It is now up to the public authorities to see to it that the large population is fed, for everyone knows that without adequate diet no community can remain healthy."

Medicine in the year 2000 will be more prophylactic than therapeutic; it has been so since the beginning of the century. Before investigating new antibiotics to treat tuberculosis, for example, attempts will be made to prevent it by means of good food and adequate housing for everyone.

Health and peace will be based in the future on peaceful and benevolent coexistence with germs and political opponents, independent of chemotherapies or atomic bombs. Disease prevention through conditions that improve physical and mental health—pure air, wholesome food—will lead to healthier minds and clearer thinking, which in turn may contribute to a world peace based on love for life and the absence of fear. Wars are conceived in men's brains before they are fought on the battlefield. The healthy, happy men of the future may create a peaceful, happy world.

VI. The integration of antibiotic culture.

In conclusion, let us consider the last aspect of the clinical case history—its educational value—and let us also consider the need for integrating the knowledge we derive from it.

The enormous importance of antibiotic therapy in the present-day clinical case history of an infectious patient indicates that a new branch of medicine has been created: antibiotic science. Antibiotic medicine has grown so rapidly that it already represents a doctrinal corpus of considerable scientific importance.

One of the principal tasks of the physician in the next half century will be to achieve in antibiotic medicine what living matter achieves teleologically in biology.

As unicellular organisms become multicellular and their vital structure becomes more complicated, a growing functional differentiation is created that requires the integration of all these functions within the unity of the biologic whole that is an organism. Similarly, in the field of science the growing differentiation of knowledge requires also an organic integration to co-ordinate all the aspects of a given doctrinal corpus under formation.

The need of integrating scientific know-how in antibiotic medicine requires that this branch of medical science be inspired by the same desire for the integration of medicine that gave form and meaning to the life of Thomas Linacre, medical humanist and organizer of the Royal College of Physicians of London in Henry VIII's time. The humanistic genius of Thomas Linacre led him to apply in practice Roger Bacon's notion that all the sciences are related and that they are only integral parts of a great whole.

Now, the integration of knowledge is an intellectual process and as such occurs only within individuals. Therefore, the integration of what we know about antibiotic medicine has to be carried out in the mind of today's physician, so that later it may be translated into all the activities of theoretical study, scientific research, and clinical practice of his life. Toward that end, the research worker and the physician must ever keep in mind that the original meaning of the word "doctor" is *teacher*.[E]

Let us not forget that an aspect of medicine has always been predominant at each step in the historic evolution of antibiotic medicine. Antibiotic medicine began as scientific research; later it became clinical practice, and then medical teaching. Today it presents a problem of medical administration, and interest is ever-growing in the progress of means of scientific communication for the creation of a culture in the field of antibiotic medicine.

The basic tools of this culture are medical journalism, scientific literature, conventions and symposia, films, radio, and television, and everything that can be used in the field of communication to spread teaching through visual and auditory aids.

The next half century will witness a notable development in the art of communicating ideas on antibiotic medicine, translated into technical methods such as the creation of an International Institute of Antibiotics, Chairs of Antibiotic Medicine, an International Museum of the History and Development of Antibiotics, and publications for the widest diffusion of the maximum amount of practical knowledge on antibiotic medicine to the greatest number of physicians in the shortest time possible.

One of the important things to be achieved in the future is the formation of an International Collection of New Antibiotics.

In doing research today on each new compound it is necessary to ascertain whether it is a new antibiotic or not. This can be done only by comparing it in the laboratory with other antibiotics, already described, since very often chemical descriptions of new antibiotics leave much to be desired. Since it is difficult for some research workers to furnish appreciable amounts of their compounds, a central international organization should be formed to furnish research workers with samples of the substances they need, enabling them to further their task and to ascertain what antibiotic they have discovered.

Such a collection existing alongside a museum containing all the important elements—manuscripts, microscopes, culture plates—relating to the history of the development of antibiotics as well as the respective iconography, from pictures of the important men involved in the discovery and development of antibiotics to photos in electronic microscopes, might form the basis for an International Institute of Antibiotics.

The International Institute of Antibiotics would be devoted to the history, culture, and development of antibiotics and would embrace a collection of samples of new antibiotics, as well as a center of publications, films, lectures, magazines, books, and iconography on antibiotics.

These are suggestions that the pharmaceutical industry could turn into reality. The directors of this industry have already turned into reality the utopian dream of an antibiotic production fabulous both in quantity and in quality. They would cover themselves with even greater glory if they brought antibiotic culture into being by the establishment of an International Institute of Antibiotics. Such an institution would in turn create Chairs of Antibiotic Medicine throughout the world, endowing them with visual aids, such as books, magazines, inconographies, films, and television; auditive aids, such as lectures, recordings, and radio; and miscellaneous aids, such as an international collection of samples[F] to facilitate teaching, research, and practice in the next half century of antibiotic medicine.

Such integration of the various branches of antibiotic medicine into one corpus of great scientific value and practical importance would represent the crystallization of all the progress achieved in this field, which today is dedicated to the science of healing, but in the future will be dedicated to the art of preventing disease.

Gazing across the panorama of the next half century, antibiotics loom as a majestic bridge spanning not space but the endless river of Time. Over this bridge Medicine advances toward its fateful rendezvous with the Future.

It is a beautiful paradox that modern medicine owes much luster and greatness to the discovery of antibiotics. Because greatness is ideals, but it is also humility. And modern medicine has received a noble lesson in humility, for it owes its most exalted greatness to the humble, minute world of molds and microbes.

NOTES

A. Introduced by Richard Bright when he pointed out the importance of the study of urine in kidney diseases.

B. These are the Platonic and Hippocratic concepts, realist or nominalist, rationalist or empirical.

C. Greater emphasis is being put all the time on the study of the nonspecific physiologic factors governing the phenomenon of parasitism. Pasteur said that "there is a fundamental difference between disease and its predisposing causes." Herpes is a practical example—as Dubos has shown—of a human infection where, notwithstanding ancient ideas, the reaction of the body is more important than the still unknown causal agent.

D. Thanks to antibiotics, according to Dr. C. C. Tauer, Medical Adviser, National Office of Vital Statistics, Public Health Service, a million and a half lives were saved in the first 15 years of the sulfonamide and antibiotic era. These lives represent those persons who might have died if the percentage of mortality from certain infections had continued in the same proportion after 1937—when sulfonamides began to be used in the U.S.A.—as in former years. Of the lives saved from 1938 to 1952, inclusive, 1,100,000 persons would have died of pneumonia and influenza, 76,000 mothers would have died of puerperal fever, 136,000 persons of syphilis, and 90,000 of appendicitis.

E. To facilitate the ideal of the future that all physicians should be research workers, practical clinicians, and teachers, we have to stimulate that intellectual impulse toward investigation, which Bertrand Russell called "the impatience for incomplete discovery," that comes from curiosity, admiration, and reverence for ideas, man's most precious treasure. The spirit that incites the physician to consider science as the art of the improbable, just as politics is the art of the probable, is the same spirit that inspired the words *academy* and *symposium,* which since Plato's time have designated places and occasions for the communion of individual wisdoms and for the formation of a collective body of knowledge.

The university of the future will venerate these qualities, will cultivate ideas, will integrate them, purify and discipline them, lending coherence and power to the intellectual progress serving man. This intellectual advancement will make progress in the field of antibiotics possible.

F. It could be a center like the National Standards Collection in London.

ANTIBIOTICS TODAY AND
THE MEDICINE OF THE FUTURE

ignus non sum. Your graciousness explains my presence here as moderator of the discussions at this symposium, which for two days will turn Manhattan into a nervous center of international scientific thought. The honor you have conferred upon me really belongs to the journal with which I am associated, *Antibiotics & Chemotherapy,* a leader in the antibiotic crusade in which I am but a participant.

I would like to extend greetings to the distinguished authorities in public health who have come here from the four corners of the earth and who are dedicated to the fulfillment of a noble task and a historic mission. It is my privilege to be bound to many of you by a common Latin background and by the golden thread of our native language; it is an even greater privilege to be bound to all of you by that cultural and academic brotherhood which is one of the sturdiest columns supporting the science of tomorrow.

I would also like to extend greetings to the Lederle Laboratories, who have organized this great symposium in which we witness the union of science and conscience, of professional co-operation and the spiritual affinities of distinguished men of science from many great countries. This is one more valuable contribution to be added to the many already made by the Lederle Laboratories toward the progress of pharmaceutical chemistry and clinical medicine as well as toward the crystallization of an ideal of service to physicians throughout the world.

Delivered at the International Symposium on Antibiotics, New York, November 2–3, 1954.

If universities and hospitals represent the scientific consciousness of a nation, the laboratories of pharmaceutical companies represent its scientific subconscious. And—as I have said elsewhere, and please forgive the sin of self-quotation for which even Dante could not find an adequate punishment— ". . . just as the authentic truth about man emanates from his unconscious mind in the form of dreams and inspirations, so does many a great truth responsible for notable progress in science emanate from this scientific subconscious of a nation represented by pharmaceutic laboratories. And just as in an iceberg the most important part is invisible under the water, so in the field of antibiotics the most important part is constituted by the invisible research workers in the pharmaceutical industry, who have anonymously contributed some of the most notable discoveries in this field." [1]

CLASSICAL AND ROMANTIC MODERATORS

If nothing else, my words express my emotion, that hormone of the soul without which nothing has any meaning. I have full confidence in the work of this symposium. If we marry simplicity to fervor, understanding to clarity, and idealism to common sense, and if we bring the teachings of the past to bear upon the experience of the present, we shall help unveil the mysteries of the future.

Dictionaries tell us that the word "moderator," the role I play here, comes from the Latin *moderare,* meaning "to maintain within certain limits." Fortunately, for me, your knowledge and wisdom will make such a duty unnecessary. The brilliant array of authorities present here is sufficient guarantee that every one of us will learn a great deal about antibiotic problems. I am only too eager to listen to what you have to tell us and shall therefore limit myself at this juncture to tracing some black and white outlines showing how the antibiotics of today may influence the medicine of tomorrow.

The moderator of a symposium can use the floor in two ways: to help the audience give concrete form to their thoughts, which is the classical way; or to encourage them to widen the cultural horizon of their ideas, which is the romantic way. As I would not presume to employ the classical way with such a brilliant audience, I shall instead encourage you to think about the philosophic significance of antibiotics and to realize the impact they may have on the medicine of the future.

ANTIBIOTICS AND PUBLIC HEALTH

Your main concern—and I am now addressing our illustrious foreign colleagues—is problems of public health, problems I coped with in Spain some years ago and which still command my greatest interest and devotion.

To grasp the impact that antibiotics are having on public health, we must keep in mind that the last few years have witnessed a tremendous philosophic change in the mission of medicine and the role of the physician.[A]

The physician began in history as a witch doctor; he became a priest among the geometric white marble forms of the temples of Aesculapius; he donned the philosopher's toga as the Renaissance sun, filtering through stained-glass windows, shed multicolored patterns on the floors of cathedrals and universities; and finally he became a scientist only in the last half of the nineteenth century.

MEDICINE MEN AND MEN OF MEDICINE

Since the beginning of history, the physician has been the *man who heals*.[2] This he did in primitive times through magic and sorcery; later, through natural resources based on a healthy Hippocratic criterion; today, through scientific medicine.

The difference between primitive magic medicine and today's scientific medicine is that the former was concerned with the *who*, the *where*, and the *when:* the person doing the healing, the place of healing, and the time of healing; while scientific medicine is concerned only with the *what* and the *how:* the drug and how it acts. Magic medicine claimed that its effects derived from the magnetic powers of the medicine man, who could be successful only in a given place chosen by the gods or the demons, and only under certain favorable positions of the sun, the moon, and other heavenly constellations. Scientific medicine is not concerned with the physician's race, religion, appearance, or personality, so long as he uses the appropriate remedy (the *what*) and knows why this remedy should heal the patient (the *how*).

The physician is also the *man who knows*. Through his knowledge he contributes to the progress of culture and civilization, and his knowledge reflects the state of art, culture, and philosophy in his time. He enriches man's knowledge of himself.

The physician is the *man who can foretell* future events. He can predict the course of an illness, anticipate the course of an epidemic that might change the fate of a nation, and prophesy the future of a human being by studying his physical and mental constitution, his habits, forebears, and illnesses. The physician is the prophet of the individual history of man and, to a certain extent, of the psychobiologic history of nations. In this sense, the physician engaged in public health is the prophet of our times who may, in the future when new means are available, foretell and even prevent almost all diseases.

Finally, the physician is an *organizer of human life*. He contributes to the improvement of man's home, his clothes, food, habits, amusements, reading, laws, and institutions. Considered from this angle, the physician's work is the cornerstone of the historical destiny of man.

THE BIRTH AND DEVELOPMENT OF PREVENTIVE MEDICINE

As we proceed from the particular to the general, from the changes in the physician's role to the changes in medicine, we must remember that the history of medicine is the story of a gigantic conflict between dogmatic tradition and free thinking, authority and experimentation, conformism and renovation. But the most important events in the evolution of medicine took place in the last fifty years, as the art of healing gradually became a science of prevention.

In the golden age of Periclean Greece, medicine was merely *techne iatrike,* while in imperial Rome, when Galen flourished, medicine was *ars medendi*. Only under the influence of certain currents of ideas, as Henry Sigerist recently pointed out,[3] such as the Platonic ideal of *kalokathia* or the development of individuals sound in mind and body, or Quintillian's ideal of *homo Ciceronianus* as the intellectual model of adolescence, did the first signs of preventive medicine appear.

Preventive measures, such as the tragic isolation imposed on lepers, who were literally buried alive in their sackcloth robes and sinister masks, or on pregnant women and people suffering from certain diseases, came to the fore sporadically. Such passive medicine, based exclusively on *isolation,* was followed by a truly *curative* medicine that considered the patient as an individual.

Our era is witnessing the rise to power of preventive medicine. As medical research advances, with the aid of new instruments we discover the secrets of diseased human anatomy; as the horizon of the human eye expands with the use of the electron microscope and we discover microbes hitherto invisible, we become more and more concerned with the causes of disease and their prevention. We go even further. Just as we have been replacing the old concept of a *people* as an isolated ethnic group with that of a *nation,* that is to say, a people with a universal function, so do we now think of the patient not only as an *individual* but also as a *person,* that is, an individual with a social function.

Medicine today is concerned with the individual, sick or healthy, and with the society to which he belongs; its ideal objectives are to prevent illness in human society and to help in the patient's readjustment to that society. This means that the physician must accept a greater social and moral responsibility toward his fellow men and must add to his scientific knowledge other facts drawn from medical history, sociology, and economics.

Every day the physician acquires greater insight into society as a configuration of social groups and into the different problems of public hygiene with which each group has to contend. Furthermore, the physician attempts to put into practice the concept of rehabilitation, of the patient's readaptation to society, because he knows that a human being is not cured of his illness so long as he cannot return to society as an active member within the limit of his aptitudes. That is why in our world, a world threatened by atomic holocausts, the physician who attempts, individually or through public health organizations, to transmute the new discoveries of science into human values adds a new seal of glory to medicine. For our profession is among the very few with eyes constantly trained on the improvement of human conditions in general.[B]

THE GOALS OF THE MEDICINE OF THE FUTURE

Modern medicine has five main objectives that trace the simple but gigantic outline of the medicine of the future: (1) to maintain the health of the individual and of the community through adequate education in hygiene and the adoption of the necessary public health measures; (2) to prevent disease, particularly contagious disease, through the organization of special services by departments of public health and similar organizations for the protection of the health of the community, especially of children and pregnant women, and through the promotion of industrial medicine and mental hygiene education; (3) to establish public services to cope with individual and collective disease, such as epidemics and wartime casualties, thus combining medicine, economic sociology, and sanitary measures; (4) to rehabilitate the patient by returning him to such work as will not endanger his health; and (5) to protect the life and health of the aged.

To accomplish this vast program successfully, the physician, the research worker, and the teacher must co-operate with one another and with hospitals, universities, and departments of public health. Only then will physicians, as professionals, approximate the Homeric ideal of being like gods, while as men, they will be "only a little lower than the angels." (Psalms 8:5.)

Let us not forget that the history of the human being is a constant struggle against oblivion. The incandescent nucleus of man's personality is an irrepressible desire for immortality. Since biologic immortality is unattainable, man attempts to master his environment and to perpetuate himself through art or a discovery or some other accomplishment, or simply through his family. But there are two great forces that constantly threaten man with destruction and the oblivion of premature death—war and disease. War he cannot prevent, since he has not succeeded yet in organizing a psychologic medicine for such a purpose; disease he tries to overcome through preventive medicine. If successful, he will achieve not Faust's eternal youth but certainly a long life rich in creative achievement.

In many countries diseases caused by filth have been eliminated. Romantic visions of the Crusaders marching to Jerusalem with drums beating, banners flying, and swords sparkling; of medieval castles with proud crenelated towers, imposing panoplies, rich tapestries, silks, hounds, pages, jousts, and tournaments; of the court of Louis XIV with sun-drenched arbors, courtiers and lovely ladies bedecked in fabrics more brilliant than the peacocks in their gardens—none of these should crowd out the fact that beneath the resplendent armor of the Crusader swarmed a myriad of insects and microbes, carriers of horrible plagues; that the dripping walls of castles enclosed a Goya-like phantasmagoria of filth in bedroom and kitchen; that the bodies of lords and ladies alike were covered with pustules; that the dwellings of the serfs were more pigsties than homes; that at the royal courts, which we admire so much in the paintings of Watteau, Boucher, and Fragonard, people covered their pock-marked faces with all sorts of cosmetics; that perfumes disguised the stench of ill-washed bodies; and that beneath lace and silk the skin harbored every type of contagious disease.

Today, civilized nations have eliminated such horrible living conditions. With the aid of antibiotics, chemotherapeutics, hormones, vitamins, and other drugs, human life has been prolonged from the average of twenty-five years for the child of the fifteenth century to sixty years for American children. Of course, although antibiotics, serums, and vaccines have rescued man from childhood diseases and hold out to him a good probability of reaching maturity, we are still faced with such diseases of maturity as heart conditions, arteriosclerosis, cancer, and mental illnesses, all of which are constantly increasing. And we know very little about how to prolong life beyond the established limits of old age.

ANTIBIOTICS AND THE MAINTENANCE OF HEALTH

Let us now examine the impact of antibiotics on the five great objectives of the medicine of the future.

First of all, antibiotics have had a considerable effect on the *maintenance of health*. In agriculture they have served to stimulate the development and growth of animals to an extent hitherto unknown; and only a short time ago several research workers at Western Reserve University reported on the use of a broad-spectrum antibiotic, mixed in small doses with food, to stimulate the development and growth of undernourished children.

Closely allied with this is the use of antibiotics as *preventives* wherever the danger of infectious disease exists. In schools, antibiotics have enabled physicians to combat successfully the imminence of epidemics and to protect sick children from serious infectious complications. Antibiotics have also helped to prevent heart lesions after rheumatic fever, complications of the renal septic foci, and bronchopulmonary complications in other infections. The carrier phase in many infectious diseases has also been eliminated, and localized tonsillar and pharyngeal infections have been prevented from spreading. In the armed forces, certain chemotherapies have warded off the threat of malaria and other tropical diseases, while the preventive use of antibiotics has minimized the risk of venereal disease, that scourge of mankind that dates back to the time when Mars first became interested in Venus' shapely torso. The use of antibiotics in battlefield hospitals has made it easier for physicians to perform emergency surgery on the wounded; and, in combination with rapid helicopter transportation to rear-line hospitals (as happened in Korea), antibiotics have prevented many postoperative infections. Antibiotics have also helped diminish mortality from traumatisms and civilian accidents, thereby reducing absenteeism in industry.

ANTIBIOTICS IN CLINICAL MEDICINE

So far we have spoken of antibiotics as curative agents in infections. In a speech delivered several days ago in Washington, D. C.,[4] I mentioned how antibiotics have altered the picture of clinical medicine.[c]

Antibiotics have radically changed the natural history of many diseases. Sydenham mentioned symptoms and signs of diseases that were modified by medicines. Antibiotics have so changed the picture of many diseases that if we compare a clinical history of pneumonia in Hippocrates' time with one in Osler's day we shall see that scarcely any difference exists in the clinical picture and the course of the fever; but if we compare a clinical history of pneumonia made twenty years ago with one made today, we would see how utterly dissimilar they are, especially the fever. The same could be said about other infections.

Heinrich Berg[5] has pointed out that classical hematology considered the blood picture to be the essential guiding factor in diagnosis. But this picture does not hold up when antibiotics are prescribed in aggressive doses. In his presidential address at the opening of the Swiss Congress of Medicine in 1953, Alder deplored that very fact in the following statements: "Diseases usually associated with leukocytosis have lost that guiding symptom. The characteristic count of leukocytes in our medical treatises now belongs to history; overnight they have been eliminated without any consideration." In other words, as the natural history of diseases is changed by antibiotics, medical tradition loses its value at the bedside of the patient.

Antibiotics are therefore transforming all three aspects of medicine: the *clinical* aspect, as the physician is obliged to use new drugs and techniques; *research,* as new light is shed on the philosophic concept of disease, its prevention, and treatment; and *teaching,* as the changes in the natural history of infections, epidemiology, and medical geography radically change the facts taught in universities.

ANTIBIOTICS AND THE REHABILITATION OF PATIENTS

In the Medicine of the Future the objective of rehabilitation will be closely related to the effect of antibiotics on the different clinical entities. By abbreviating the course of infections, eliminating complications, simplifying treatment so that it may be administered even at home, and by frequently checking contagiousness, antibiotics are causing a revolution in the field of rehabilitation.

Treating the patient at home decongests hospitals, leaves more beds free for patients suffering from diseases not yet curable, shortens the course of infections, and reduces the number of working days lost due to sickness, thereby increasing industrial output. Reducing the danger of contagion permits a faster readaptation of patients to family and social environments, and, even more important, rapid antibiotic therapy cuts down long, painful, and costly treatments, making the economic factor less important in the prognosis of certain diseases.

Let us dwell a while on this point and compare the panorama of two diseases as they bear on the economic aspects of the treatment. In the case of cancer, the only difference between a rich and a poor patient is that the rich patient can afford more medical attention and costly palliative medication. But if the tumor is malignant, both patients are unfortunately condemned to die, and the difference in economic status will mean nothing. In diseases like tuberculosis, however, the introduction of antibiotics, isoniazid, and other chemotherapeutic agents represents a major change. Formerly the treatment of both wealthy and poor patients was, barring certain unimportant drugs, essentially the therapy recommended by Hippocrates two thousand years ago: fresh air, rest, and nourishing food. The poor patient, who could not follow this elementary but costly advice, had fewer chances of recovery than the wealthy patient. Antibiotics have, in the main, leveled this difference and grant both types of patient the same right to be cured and perhaps to return to a normal life.

The entire picture, indeed the entire structure of our social life, has changed, and this calls for a redirection of thought and action.

ANTIBIOTICS AND GERONTOLOGY

We now come to the last vital objective of the Medicine of Tomorrow: the prolongation of healthy, happy old age by adding life to years and years to life. The question is: what will medicine do with the lives it is saving and the new society of old people it is helping to develop? Gerontology is already studying this problem, but the Medicine of Tomorrow cannot escape its responsibility.[D]

Antibiotic medicine will no doubt eliminate some of the common infections that formerly shortened the life expectancy of old people; it will cure small infections that render old age difficult and unhappy, and it may even contribute to the general maintenance of health in advanced age. As the proportion of old people increases, chronic, degenerative, and crippling diseases will also increase. Since the diseases of childhood, adolescence, and youth are mainly of an infectious nature, they will probably be eliminated through appropriate prophylaxis. The enemy of the early years of a person's life is external; it is a threat *from without*—infections, traumatisms—and we know how to deal with it. The enemy of the mature years comes *from within*—stress, psychoses, cancer, heart disease—and we have not yet discovered its prophylaxis. By overcoming infections, which, like a curtain of fire, threaten to cut off life at its early stages, antibiotics are forcing medicine to conquer degenerative diseases.

But the Medicine of Tomorrow has another mission: to shape social structure so that man's hidebound division of years into youth, maturity, and old age will allow for a dynamic maturity, an active old age, and a peaceful senility, after which he may serenely follow the path to the land of shadows.

Of course, all this means a larger world population, which in turn demands a greater food production. Antibiotics are helping in three different ways to increase the production of animal proteins, so valuable nutritionally to man: first, as pesticides with a remarkable phytotherapeutic effect, they prevent or cure plagues that destroy not only the food so necessary for animals but also valuable vegetable and plant life of great value to man; second, in veterinary medicine, they prevent and cure many animal diseases, thereby increasing the possibility of animals reaching an age at which they have greater value on the world food market; and third, as a supplement in small quantities to animal diet, they stimulate growth.

Antibiotics Today and the Medicine of the Future 51

Not only have antibiotics accelerated the rhythm of all aspects of medicine—diagnosis, prognosis, and therapy—but they have also hastened scientific research. There still are people who deplore the fact that medicine, especially in the field of antibiotics, is proceeding too quickly. I confess that I love haste, a deliberate, prudent haste, the *festina lente* of the ancient Romans, the haste to fulfill one's duties well and promptly.[6]

I love the haste of those who hurry because they know that there is a great deal to be done and little time to do it, of those who drive themselves even though they know that they will never reach the end because the road of science has no end. One should hurry to do things only to keep on doing more.

When haste is an anguish to finish in order to begin all over again, it is a creative haste. The anguish of life is action in search of being. The man who makes haste longs to do something great in his limited lifespan.

THE LANGUAGE OF SCIENCE

I should like to add a few words about the language used at meetings like this one.

A common language is the strongest bond between nations. A common language makes England, Australia, Canada, and the United States stand together in historical crises. Sharing the memory of Romeo's gentle words or Hamlet's melancholy meditations, whether they are read in Plymouth, Miami, Sydney, or Ontario, makes it possible for several countries to conceive of economic interrelations under a common banner of ideals and interests; just as the voice of Don Quixote, Cervantes' mad, pure, romantic knight, provides a community of interests for Spanish-speaking peoples.

But when peoples do not speak the same language and cannot exchange ideas verbally, they must resort to some other medium if they wish to draw closer. The language of science recognizes no frontiers, no barriers. It unites all men in one common crusade: the search for truth, the progress of science.

When a scientist, whatever his nationality, approaches a foreign colleague on the subject of antibiotics, clinical problems, or public health, such semantic difficulties as may exist between them are overcome by the brotherhood of their goal and their dreams. That is why I believe that at meetings such as this one we are weaving the splendrous tapestry of the medicine of tomorrow, not with words but with strands of light emanating from present-day medical knowledge.

I conclude, therefore, reiterating my faith in symposiums such as this one, which endeavor to strengthen scientific spirit and to reconcile art and science in medicine and in clinical and sociologic research. For just as those ancient vases containing the hearts of great heroes stood as symbols of gallantry and noble deeds, so does this symposium stand as a symbol of the scientific dreams and hopes of the thirty-six nations represented here.

Let us shout in all directions our desire to create an all-embracing preventive medicine, in the hope that our voices will reach the four corners of the earth and commit all men of science to a vow of universal brotherhood. It is this solemn vow that history demands of us as a guarantee for a future greater than ever for medicine.

NOTES

A. *En passant,* it would be of interest to point out what Douglas Guthrie recently and brilliantly observed,[7] namely, that today we know only a little more than our ancestors did about the basic concept of disease. The primitive medicine man knew two types of disease: those caused by a demon entering the body, and those produced by the soul leaving the body. He expelled the demons with potions and retrieved the soul through exorcisms. Today we call the invading demons bacteria and overcome them with antibiotics; and we call lost souls "complexes" and retrieve them through psychoanalysis.

The basic philosophy being the same, the physician today joins hands with the primitive medicine man when he shoulders a social responsibility toward his patient. I think Virchow put it very well a hundred years ago when he said: "Medicine is a social science . . . anthropology in its widest sense . . . and its supreme task is to see that society rests on a firm physiological basis."

B. The importance of maintaining human health as the ideal goal of medicine is in fact emphasized in the preamble to the Constitution of the World Health Organization: "The enjoyment of the highest attainable standard of health is one of the fundamental rights of every human being without distinction of race, religion, political belief, economic or social condition."

This is the foundation that supports the majestic structure of preventive medicine, which in turn foreshadows the medicine of the future.

C. Antibiotics have revolutionized the concept of the nature of disease. Sydenham's concept of disease as *species morbosa* has been replaced by the modern etiologic nosology, which is the basis of the causal thought prevalent in medicine today. In addition, antibiotics have created a *clinical* bacteriology and a *clinical* pharmacology. Furthermore, as they focused the physician's attention on the specific bacteriologic problem involved in each disease, they taught him that the *location* of a germ is what determines to a great extent the resultant lesion.

Antibiotics have again drawn attention to disease in general and to the specific disease of the patient, i.e., to the generic disturbance as found in textbooks *and* to the particular malady found at the patient's bedside. The physician has been obliged not only to study the patient clinically, but also to subject him to laboratory tests to determine the characteristics of his particular disease as a representative case of a generic disease.

Antibiotics have also forced us to reappraise our ideas on the toxicity of therapeutic agents, reminding us of the forgotten pharmacologic truth that toxic agents are often the most active, and that the important thing is not to reject an antibiotic because it is toxic but to attempt to reduce its toxicity or to direct it exclusively at the microbe.

Antibiotics have radically changed the picture of surgery and of medical specialties. The physician today is no longer only a *minister Naturae*, that is, a servant of nature who tries to aid her by favoring the natural processes of suppuration, repair, and cicatrization of wounds; the physician today is a *magister Naturae* who supplements the natural processes with his own knowledge, casting legions of "friendly" germs into the battlefield to destroy "enemy" germs and making allies of microbes that were formerly fearsome.

Among the most important contributions made by antibiotics to clinical medicine and to surgery today, there stands out the preoperative treatment of tuberculosis with streptomycin, isoniazid, para-aminosalicylic acid, and other chemotherapeutic agents. The result has been a widening of the scope of operative collapsotherapy (extrapleural pneumothorax and thoracoplasty) and pulmonary resections, reducing complications such as empyemas, bronchopulmonary fistulas, and hematogenous disseminations.

Antibiotics have accelerated progress in bone and joint surgery and have improved prognosis and therapeutics in orthopedics and traumatology, including burns by atomic radiations; and in neurosurgery, they have made possible treatment of the surgical septic processes of the central nervous system; they are also important prophylactics in plastic surgery, proctology, and pediatrics, and are very valuable in infectious complications in obstetrics, otologic, odontologic, and ophthalmologic surgery.

The bold but provocative hypothesis has been advanced that antibiotics, acting as alarmogens throughout the pituitary-adrenal system through the mechanism of Selye's general adaptation syndrome, may play a still unexplored role in the state of health, just as they play an important role in the diseased state. We *do* know that antibiotics are capable of changing the anatomic, radiologic, clinical, and immunobiologic picture of a disease as well as the causal germ; they must therefore also change the patient's anatomophysiologic picture.

D. From the second World War on, antibiotics have been greatly responsible for the increase in the proportion of people of advanced age in the United States. The total population of the United States has doubled since 1900, with a fourfold increase in the number of people older than 65. In their interesting study of this subject, Pratt and Dufrenoy[8] state that this disproportion is partly due to antibiotics. In 1900, pneumonia caused the death of 159 persons out of 100,000; today the ratio is only 12 out of 100,000. The number of deaths from tuberculosis decreased from 181 per 100,000 in 1900 to 20 out of the same number today; and death from Rocky Mountain fever decreased from a proportion of 40 to 50 per cent ten years ago to almost nothing today.

The present population of the world is about 2500 millions; by 1960 it may increase to 3636 millions. Four billion human beings, say the agriculture and food experts, are the most the earth can accommodate. To the increased lifespan, which has reached 60 years for both sexes, we must add the reduction in mortality from childhood diseases and acute and chronic infectious diseases such as tuberculosis, malaria, syphilis, frambesia, intestinal parasitosis, and leprosy (there are still about 350 millions suffering from malaria and about five million lepers, altogether a quarter of the total population of the planet).[9]

As antibiotics eradicate "old" diseases, they make room for "new" ones. Infections, in the form of those vaguely termed "fevers," represented 75 per cent of all medical cases in Thomas Sydenham's times; today, except for epidemics, they represent a mere 5 per cent in this country. Years ago, infection caused the death of 25 per cent of all human beings. Today, consumptive and degenerative diseases, with the diseases of old age, are the principal causes of death. This means that an ever-diminishing population of young people will have to guarantee the existence of an ever-increasing population of old people.

The solution to the problem will depend more and more on the recognition of the fact that time is relative not only in Einstein's theories but in our daily lives. In contrast with the classic concept of physical and chronologic time, we are confronted with the modern concept of Lecomte de Nouy's *biologic time* buttressed by the use of antibiotics.[10] This concept stems from the idea that age may be measured in physiologic terms instead of in years. Physiologically, many people today are younger than their parents and grandparents were at the same chronologic age. Antibiotics contribute to guaranteeing this historic prolongation of youth. Only the years will tell, however, whether the prolongation of an individual's youth is not paid for by the acceleration of the aging of the species.

IN QUEST OF THE BROAD SPECTRUM

L ife is an awe-inspiring biologic symphony made possible by the activity of certain symbiotic bacteria indispensable to human life (for instance, the intestinal flora bacteria, whose symbiotic action produces certain substances necessary for hematopoiesis); but there are also pathogenic germs, and against these deadly enemies man has developed a rich and powerful chemotherapeutic arsenal. For more than two thousand years, from Hippocrates to Pasteur, man tried to fight infection with magical and empirical weapons. In the beginning he attempted to expel the causal agents of infection— regarded at first as demons, later as miasmas, and finally as germs— by means of prayers, herbs, or the magic metals of Paracelsus, the founder of medicinal chemistry. Next, man progressed to the point of attacking infectious diseases with serums and vaccines, thus reinforc- ing the natural organic defenses. And then, one memorable day in the history of medicine, a French veterinarian threw the window open and let in the light of the microbial doctrine of infection.

If, according to the age-old saying, all roads lead to Rome, all paths in bacteriology lead to Pasteur. The work done by Pasteur (1822– 1895) and Koch (1843–1910) established the bases of medical microbiology. Although Pasteur did little in the field of chemotherapy, his work stimulated Lister in 1867 to do research on septic wounds, which obsessed not only him but all surgeons a century ago. Twenty years before Lister, in 1847, Semmelweis introduced the idea of dis- infecting the surgeon's hands with calcium chloride to prevent puer- peral fever. This was the beginning of the three great methods to fight infection: disinfection; antisepsis, which would later become asepsis; and chemotherapy.

In his crusade against "putrefaction" of operative wounds, Lister adopted carbolic acid sprays as his principal weapon, destroying bacteria in the air before they had a chance to reach operative wounds. This subsequently led to the use of hydrosoluble chemotherapeutic agents. Lister's antisepsis, however, was limited in scope because it allowed only for the destruction of the bacterial enemy *before* it invaded the body and penetrated the tissues. That is why such antisepsis was later replaced by asepsis, a true prophylactic chemotherapy that made use of chemical substances to treat infections that had already taken root. These substances, however, proved to be active only in superficial infections and were more toxic to the tissues than to the bacteria. But the philosophic principle that guided Lister still prevails in surgery. The sterilization of instruments avails itself of heat as a *physical* agent, but disinfection of the skin and wounds must be carried out through *chemical* agents.

About twenty years (1847–1865) elapsed between Semmelweis' and Lister's discoveries. After Lister came almost half a century of groping in the dark, until, in 1909, Ehrlich's chromotherapy with salvarsan ushered in the age of chemotherapy in bacterial infections. Ehrlich's "magic bullets," however, hit only limited targets. Twenty-five years later, Domagk introduced the sulfonamides, which enabled the physician to put the bacteria "to sleep," thus arresting their development and enabling the leukocytes to sweep them out with the brooms of their pseudopods. The sulfonamides were useful as a systemic treatment, but they showed poor results when used topically, since their powers were neutralized in those great leukocyte graveyards—the pus of septic wounds.

Six years earlier, when some humble *Penicillium* spores drifted from gray smoky skies onto a culture plate in a London hospital, there was planted—not only on the plate but in Fleming's mind—the seedling that was later to grow into the wonder crop of antibiotics.

IN QUEST OF THE BROAD SPECTRUM

The history of man's struggle against infection is one of incessant, almost agonizing, searching for a drug endowed with a broad antimicrobial spectrum. Having progressed beyond the ancient Greek dream of the universal panacea and the medieval dream of the philosopher's stone, medical researchers from Pasteur on, aware of what infection represented, applied themselves to finding a drug with a wide therapeutic range and a deep healing effect; in other words, a drug capable of curing the maximum number of infections with a minimum risk to the patient.

The pharmaceutical cavalcade that began in the middle of the last century was discouraged at first: it was thought impossible to find a drug with a broad antimicrobial spectrum, because common belief held that human and bacterial protoplasms were so similar that any chemical agent that destroyed one would necessarily harm the other. Malaria was finally and successfully treated with quinine, and syphilis with Ehrlich's arsenicals; but medical opinion was that such chemotherapy was a lucky accident and could not be applied to viral and bacterial infections. The subsequent discovery of the sulfonamides, synthetic antimalarials, and antibiotics led slowly to that ideal pharmacologic horizon of the broad antimicrobial spectrum. And when the myth of the identity of the protoplasms of human and microbial cells was finally destroyed, the dike that for so many years had obstructed the course of the mighty river of antibacterial chemistry was carried away.

Broad-spectrum antibiotics, such as oxytetracycline, represent the crystallization of man's dream of a chemotherapeutic agent that would prevent the multiplication of invading germs and would destroy them without altering the function of organic cells.

"Old" antiseptics were a form of rudimentary local chemotherapy, just as arsenicals were a specific chemotherapy; but the use of antibiotics, "substances of microbial origin endowed with antibiotic powers," [2] has expanded the horizon of the clinician: horizontally—to embrace the broad antimicrobial spectrum—and vertically—to achieve depth of effect, properties that are indispensable in any agent claiming to have a broad antimicrobial spectrum, that historical Holy Grail of the crusaders of chemotherapy.

Antibiotics, a product of the moist alchemy of the earth or of molds—those tiny gnomes of the vegetable kingdom—have had a tremendous philosophic impact on modern clinical medicine, a subject I have discussed at length on other occasions.[1, 3] The glowing dawn of the antibiotic age suffuses the sky of contemporary medicine. Present antibiotic therapy affords us a glimpse of the end of the historical road where are inscribed, as on an honor roll, the diseases that for many a millennium have scourged humanity and that antibiotic medicine will finally vanquish.

The introduction of antibiotics, especially of the broad-spectrum antibiotics, has had three important consequences in modern clinical medicine: it has altered classic pathology; it has changed clinical diagnosis from pathogenic to etiologic; it has simplified anti-infectious therapy.

ALTERATION OF CLASSIC PATHOLOGY

Antibiotics have altered classic pathology because the process of disease, including infection, is a mutable reality which, like every living thing, evolves spontaneously. Sometimes, as occurs in infections, because disease depends on living species, it is subject to the same changes and degenerations as the causative germs; furthermore, because disease is a parasitic reality of human life, it, in time, evolves along with human life itself, especially because of the persistent action of drugs and the highly effective hygienic measures of present-day therapeutics.

Because antibiotics intervene in the most subtle phases of metabolism and in the most delicate enzymatic actions of bacterial life, they provoke changes in the bacteria's biologic cycle that have already been translated into radical changes in the diseases the bacteria cause. Antibiotics have influenced the natural history of such infections as syphilis, which nowadays, even when not treated with antibiotics, follows its course without the old phagedenic ulcers, and typhoid fever, which now rarely presents the splenomegalies of the old classic form.

NEW ETIOLOGIC ORIENTATION OF MEDICINE

Antibiotics have changed the concept of diagnosis in clinical medicine. Twenty years ago medical teachers and students everywhere were still overawed by the infinite variations in the subtle arts of clinical exploration, percussion, and auscultation. They delighted in lingering over the pathogenesis of a disease; they had plenty of time to debate the differential diagnosis of a syndrome, and they elaborated on the localization of the disease with the painstaking precision with which an Oriental miniaturist places specks of color on his miniatures.

Today pathogenesis is more and more considered as a stopping-off point on the way to the great terminal station of etiology. Modern medicine is constantly becoming more etiologic in its conceptions, more dynamic in its specific therapies, even at the sacrifice of the rigid precision that characterized anatomic localizations and clinical descriptions in textbooks at the beginning of our century.

But the symptom in itself, its nuances and qualities, is not important, for paradoxically the only thing normal in clinical pathology is its abnormality. That is why it is of the utmost importance to consider rapidly the vast mural of syndromes and symptoms in clinical pathology and then proceed to discover the secret of its etiology, without which therapeutics today would be as empirical as they were in the times of Avicenna.

Today, we accept the indestructible unity of the entire organism and the physiologic correlation between all organic processes, much more apparent in disease than in health. When an organ or system is ill, the entire body suffers. Recognition of that fact forces the physician

MEN, MOLDS, AND HISTORY

in our age of specialization to widen his clinical education. Modern techniques give greater breadth and depth to his control of the disease process. Even as he focuses therapy on the specific cause of the disease, the modern physician learns all he can about general medicine, because his therapy is guided by that "etiologic preoccupation" which is tantamount to his wish to treat the entire organism.

This new etiologic orientation of medicine has led to the *etiologic sign,* replacing both the *lesional sign* of former anatomic pathology and the *functional sign* of physiopathology. This new etiologic sign is sometimes evident in the demonstration of the immunobiologic reaction to the invasion of an infectious agent (Widal's reaction in typhoid, Wassermann's reaction in syphilis) or in the direct observation of the causative agent (sight of the *Mycobacterium* in sputum or of the Klebs-Löffler bacillus in a tonsillar pseudomembrane).

SIMPLIFICATION OF ANTIMICROBIAL THERAPY

The third result of the introduction of antibiotics is the marvelous simplification of antimicrobial therapy. To realize this, we only have to compare the voluminous pathology treatises of fifty years ago, describing at length innumerable empirical treatments of infections, with their modern counterpart, a single chapter in a medical textbook explaining with great sparsity of words and naked statistics, aligned like shivering recruits, what specific drugs are to be used and in what dosage.

Therapy thus based on the use of antibiotics is becoming more and more etiologic and less pathogenic. It begins with the knowledge of the clinical facts, but instead of stopping as it did formerly with the pathogenic link of the pathologic process, it attempts to reach the etiology quickly. For any treatment founded only on pathogenesis is neither scientific nor acceptable practically unless the etiology is known. But even in such cases it is preferable to use antibiotics in an attempt to "focus" the group of etiologies in which the specific causal agent of the infection might be found. If after that we still do not have even a vague idea of the causative agent, it is still preferable to accept what has been called an "etiologic purpose," which serves to guide the clinician just as the stars guide the navigator without a compass.*

FACETS OF THE TETRACYCLINES

Among the broad-spectrum antibiotics, the tetracyclines deserve

---

* Quite often, paradoxically, the physician cures an infectious process of indeterminate origin with antibiotics, and such an empirical cure leads *a posteriori* to the discovery of the unknown etiology: thus he acquires a knowledge that he can apply to similar cases in the future.

In Quest of the Broad Spectrum 61

special attention for several reasons, of which the main ones are their numerous clinical indications and therapeutic successes.

Unlike penicillin, the tetracyclines were discovered not by one man but by a team of men. If in the history of medicine the discovery of certain drugs stems from the observation of Nature as a philosophic revelation of God, the discovery of these particular drugs is the result of the scientific labor of a group of investigators for whom medical art and medical science were the true revelations of man.

The discovery of the tetracyclines was not one of those "famous accidents" so frequent in medical history. These, by the way, happen only to those who deserve them, to those who possess, as Sir Henry Dale said, "natural aptitude, skilled curiosity, and mature experience." We can trace them from Archimedes' discovery of the adulteration of gold in the royal crown to Pasteur's accidental discovery of the crystallography of the two isomeric forms of tartaric acid. The discovery of the tetracyclines, on the contrary, represented the final goal of carefully planned research, in which the element of chance was reduced to a minimum by exercising maximum effort to assure the scientific precision of the project.

With the tetracyclines the term "broad spectrum" was definitely incorporated into medical terminology, and today it has spread to other clinical fields. It has been said that the broader the spectrum of an antibacterial substance the lesser its specificity and the greater its toxicity, for the most powerful broad-spectrum antibiotic theoretically would be the one that is a general protoplasmic poison. But this is not applicable to the broad-spectrum antibiotics used today by the physician, because their main characteristic is that the breadth of their antimicrobial spectrum is linked with the lowest possible toxicity spectrum. The "toxic" horizon of antibiotics like the tetracyclines is almost exclusively occupied by microbes that are susceptible to them and not by their human host.

Along with other broad-spectrum antibiotics, the tetracyclines have passed through the historical phases of isolation of their active principle, purification, stabilization, and determination of their atomic architecture which is the key to their therapeutic action against given bacterial organisms.

It is interesting that in the evolution of the tetracyclines the knowledge of their index of therapeutic activity preceded that of their chemical structure. But as soon as the latter was known, research workers tried to alter the molecular structure hoping to discover a variation in therapeutic activity.

The progress of research in this field is limited not only by the imagination of the chemist, but also by the material possibility of translating his mental conceptions into chemical realities in the laboratory. Yet it is possible to predict that future investigators will explore bacterial physiology and metabolism for the purpose of synthesizing new antibiotics specifically oriented against certain bacteria, keeping in mind, however, what phase of bacterial physiology they intend to attack, what weak points of their enzyme systems they want to alter, what bacterial metabolites they plan to replace: in short, in what way they can deliver a mortal blow to bacterial development by using the peculiar chemical structure of an antibiotic synthesized for that very purpose.

There are two phases through which the study of the effectiveness of a new therapeutic agent evolves in history. Alongside reports on isolated individual cases—so useful when one is clinically trying out a new antibiotic or an "old" one in a new group of indications—stand reports presenting the evaluation of great numbers of cases.

The first reports represent the *individual* phase of the evaluation of a drug, in which each and every result is weighed and related to the modality of each clinical case; and the second group of reports represents the *statistical* phase in which great numbers of "depersonalized" cases are used. The integration of both phases—the first dealing with individualized cases of medical practice and the second with hospital statistics—culminates in the final evaluation of an antibiotic, later translated into the formation of a doctrinal and practical corpus around it.

Attention is drawn to the increasing simplicity with which the cases and their treatment are presented in this field. The practical, even naturalistic, focus of the current reports on antibiotics confirms what Darwin said in the final years of his life: that the naturalist who counts the leaves of a plant does more to fulfill his duty to study nature than the author of purely theoretical disquisitions. From this point of view, it is of the utmost importance that we continue to compile "common" clinical histories, those "ordinary" cases that are the small change of medicine, but that, as with all small change, can be accumulated into a treasure of clinical knowledge.

ANTIBIOTICS AND THE ART OF HEALING

Broad-spectrum antibiotics have not only widened the therapeutic horizon of the physician, they have also broadened his philosophic conception of the ends, means, and resources of clinical medicine. If the second half of the nineteenth century was fertile in doctrinal elaborations, the first half of our century has reaped a magnificent therapeutic crop.

Parallel to the progress of medicine as a science, we have witnessed the rise of the art of healing per se. And healing is the most important goal not only for the patient but also for the physician. The growing splendor of experimental disciplines should not make us forget that experimentation is only an accessory of the empirical and humble, although all-important, art of healing. Only when the physician constantly bears in mind the prospects of curing his patient does he achieve true greatness for himself and for the medical profession. Paraphrasing Jorge Manrique, the classic Castilian poet, all medical knowledge, whatever course it may follow, must, like all rivers, finally flow into the vast sea of healing.

Viewed from this angle, broad-spectrum antibiotics represent a supreme contribution to the art of healing, not as an easy way of bypassing a doubtful clinical situation but as an incentive to refine diagnosis and hasten the cure of infectious diseases.

THE DRAMA OF INFECTION AND THE PATIENT AS A WHOLE

Infection is perhaps the most dramatic of man's pathologic contingencies. It mobilizes the entire organism in response to alarm warnings from those organic "Pentagons" that comprise the pituitary-adrenal axis and the hypothalamic centers. The entire organism declares war on the invading bacteria and marshals all its resources, from the most humble humoral defenses to the supreme neuroendocrine centers governing the organism. The danger is universal in any infection, and the response of the human being is also universal. Antibiotic therapy, even if specific, enjoys universality in the sense that it spreads throughout the body until it enters into battle with the bacterial invaders wherever they may be, thus also responding to that etiologic aim discussed earlier.

Antibiotic therapy is an etiologic and integral therapy, specific in its objectives and integral in its conception, as proved by the recent introduction of certain compounds combining vitamins and antibiotics, which help to fight stress in an infectious patient and to strengthen his defenses. In one word, modern therapeutic weapons are being used toward the classical goal of treating the *whole* patient.

We see, then, a restoration of the concept that the *whole* patient should be treated, including his nutrition and his psyche, even in the case of infections. Let us not forget that the word *holy* has the same etymologic root (*hal*) as the words *health* and *whole*. If medicine wishes to recover its philosophic holiness, which is the same as saying its historical dignity, it must treat the *whole* patient.

ANTIBIOTICS AND THE
PROBLEM OF MEDICAL COMMUNICATION

ANTIBIOTIC KNOWLEDGE IN TIME AND SPACE

From our various fields of clinical research and practice we are gathered here for our Fourth Annual Symposium, the object of which is to assess what progress has been made during the past year in the field of antibiotic and chemotherapeutic drugs, to consider a number of as yet unresolved clinical problems, and to outline prospects for future research. These Symposia, which started as a national experiment, have become, thanks to your efforts and work, an international institution yielding year by year an ever-increasing and bountiful harvest of rewarding discoveries.

If we look back at the three preceding Symposia and anticipate the one starting today, we can see the result of our efforts in the following figures: 580 papers; 43 new antibiotics; and more than 3600 printed pages covering the work of 1437 writers of 35 different nationalities. These figures reveal with the cold eloquence of all statistics how these Symposia have greatly increased the already considerable *corpus doctrinalis* on antibiotics, which has been growing ever since that memorable day when a patient scientist kept his rendezvous with destiny in his humble laboratory at St. Mary's Hospital in London and found the key that was to change the whole face of modern therapeutics.

Never before in the history of medicine has collaboration between clinicians and research workers devoted to the study of a single group

Delivered at the Fourth Annual Symposium on Antibiotics, Washington, D. C., October 17–19, 1956.

of curative agents produced such a monumental body of knowledge and learning. If we remember that work in other fields of therapeutics, such as alkaloids, vitamins, hormones, and serums, was developed in its beginning by isolated individuals, and later by team work, but always in a sporadic and disjointed way both in time and in space, it might strike us as remarkable that in barely fourteen years colossal progress has been made in the knowledge, research, and clinical use of as new a family of drugs as the antibiotics. This has been attained not only in time, by forcing the pace, thanks to the ever-increasing rhythm of work, of the stages of medical history, but also in space, by conducting the study of antibiotics on an international scale unprecedented in the evolution of medicine.

The headlong "vertical" progress—in time—of this work is supported by its tremendous "horizontal" expansion—in space—the result of which has been that antibiotics are now the most international of all drugs, for they may be discovered on one continent, analyzed, investigated, and developed on another, tested on still a third continent, and end up by being used in all quarters of our globe. Never has medicine been more truly historical in its scientific outlook or more universal in its horizons than in the antibiotic field.

HISTORICOPSYCHOLOGIC BACKGROUND TO THE RESEARCH ON ANTIBIOTICS IN OUR TIME

The historical reasons for the discovery of antibiotic medicine and its extraordinary progress have not hitherto been under consideration. There has never been pure chance in any discovery in the medical world, for all such events have always been tied in some way or other to the cultural atmosphere of each period, which fosters the development of certain types of discovery in preference to others. Medicine is moreover but one aspect of human endeavor, which may also manifest itself in other forms, say, literature, architecture, or music. It is therefore necessary to assess the determining factors in any particular period in the story of civilization if we wish to understand exactly the meaning of medical discoveries during such a period.

A few months from now we shall be commemorating the tercentennial of the death of William Harvey. To appreciate properly Harvey's discovery of the circulation of the blood, which changed the face of medicine after some thirteen centuries of error based on Galen's physiology, it is vital to consider the cultural atmosphere of his age, the full height of the Renaissance, in Britain and Europe. For without the sudden enthusiasm for *motion* in art, embodied in Michelangelo's work; without the triumph of the new dynamic conception of art as attested by the outburst of *chiaroscuro,* of spiraling columns that ousted the classical Greek and Roman pillars and capitals, and, above all, of baroque work that wrenched the stone of cathedrals and palaces from the mystic ecstasy of Gothic art and turned it into veritable whirlpools—without an awareness of all this, it would be impossible to understand how Harvey came to make that splendid leap from the static anatomy of Vesalius to his *Anatomia Animata,* now called physiology. And again, how he came to make his discoveries in embryology, which was another form of creating animate anatomy *in time,* just as physiology was its embodiment *in space.* The yearning to find *motion* in all forms of existence that pervaded Harvey's era, the constant mention of blood and the heart, then in vogue, as attested by Shakespeare's plays, provided the philosophic inspiration for Harvey's discovery that the blood *moves* and that it does so *in a circle.*

The increasing concentration in our time on the study of antibiotics may be considered by future historians as the philosophic expression of an age in which every effort—art, physics, science in general—was focused on disintegration, on the reduction of man and his universe to atoms. Perhaps as a reaction against the great philosophic synthesis that ruled in the eighteenth and nineteenth centuries, our own period has been inflamed with the desire to break down and analyze the infinitesimal portions of the human body, of Nature, and of the universe, a desire that has been profoundly reflected in the arts. For there is undoubtedly an obvious parallel between surrealist painting, which has split into fragments the image of man and his surroundings, nuclear physics, which has broken the universe into atoms, modern poetry, which has disjointed the rhyme and dislocated the strophe, modern architecture, which has replaced substance and solidity in building by a minimum of stone and steel to allow the outer light to enter, thus fusing the outside world with the interior hearth, and modern biochemistry, microbiology, and histopathology, which have ceased contemplating wider problems in combination and instead have focused their attention on the most minute parts of the living being and the tiniest particles of inorganic matter.

But the pendulum of History, after having traced another epoch on the clock of Eternity, will inexorably return to its starting point. Before the present century comes to an end, civilization—and, of course, in its train medicine, which is but one of its many facets— will reach back to the wider conceptions of philosophy and monumental synthesis, to a greater classicism in art and a resumption of the *integral* study of the human being in the psychologic and biologic senses, a tendency that is evident now. Antibiotics, as part of this tendency toward integration, will not be thought of merely as therapeutic agents, but all of the knowledge amassed in their study will be applied to other fields in medicine and even in allied sciences, such as agriculture, and will serve as a key to open new doors to scientific knowledge.

MEDICAL KNOWLEDGE AND MEDICAL COMMUNICATION

We have said that antibiotic medicine already has an impressive endowment of learning and theory, which is ceaselessly being renewed and increased, thanks to the efforts of clinical and laboratory researchers. This poses the problem, ever more urgent and demanding of solution, of how this tremendous amount of scientific knowledge is to be sorted, coordinated, classified, and brought under effective control.

It took three hundred years of constant labor to compile the *Corpus Hippocraticum,* which comprised the whole of the medical wisdom of the Grecian world and was a scientific instrument for physicians for more than a thousand years. Nowadays, however, the hundreds of thousands of printed pages on antibiotic medicine are only but a small portion of modern medical learning. The physician these days must also keep abreast of developments in many other areas of that vast and kaleidoscopic canvas that is our modern medical background of knowledge.

To a certain degree the body of learning in antibiotic medicine is already overrunning the time and the receptive capacity of the practicing physician. It is vital, therefore, that we organize this knowledge before it becomes a shapeless, chaotic mass, that we organize it and integrate it into a properly classified and comprehensive code. Let us therefore spend a few moments in considering the problems posed by the mass broadcast of present-day antibiotic knowledge, which is one aspect of the urgent necessity in medicine to solve without delay the problem of *medical communication.*

The goal of medical practice has been the same throughout its whole history: to cure and, if possible, to prevent disease. Medicine started as—and always will be—a *service* to mankind, the desire of one human being, the physician, to succor another human being, the patient, by helping him cure or forestall his disease. Medicine, however, was also an *art,* in that it required from the physician what every art demands, namely, a combination of imagination, feeling, skill, and experience in expressing himself artistically, which for the physician would be the satisfactory conclusion of his mission to heal. While medicine remained only a service and an art in the ancient world, medical knowledge was transmitted in the main by word of mouth, and medical teaching was imparted by master to pupil, from generation to generation, until it gradually started to take on a more permanent form when all knowledge was embodied in a *summa* or a *corpus,* such as the Hippocratic Collection, the Treatises of Galen, and the Canon of Avicenna, which were the basic tools of medical learning for more than fifteen centuries. However, not until medicine acquired the nature of a science—science requiring the objectivity of the written word as against the frequently emotional misdirection of the spoken word—to which was added the invention of the printing press, did the now fearsome problem of medical communication begin to rear its head.

The library of a physician practicing in Greece in Pericles' time consisted of a few scant ancient papyri; that of a Roman physician in the time of Tiberius of a pile of parchments of the *Corpus Hippocraticum;* that of an Arabian *hakim* practicing in Moorish Granada under the Abbasid caliphs of the Canon of Avicenna and a treatise or so of Galen's; but already in the time of Guy Patin, in seventeenth century Paris, a French physician's library contained thousands of volumes. Today, on top of all his books, the physician desirous of keeping up to date in his profession has to add the thousands of medical magazines and journals now in existence. One can well appreciate that he is faced by a frightening problem of medical communication that his ancient predecessors never knew.

THE DUTY TO COMMUNICATE

Medical communication consists of three factors: the medical information itself, be it printed, speech, or film; the author; and the reader, listener, or spectator.

We therefore recognize that transmittal of professional knowledge from one physician to others has recourse to two means: *visual*— the printed word, photographs or sketches, film or television; and *auditory*—lesson, lecture, radio talk, phonograph record, tape recording, or television.

Here we shall refer mainly to the printed word, the other means of medical communication being merely alternatives. The *word* is essential for the survival not only of science but of man himself, since without words there can be no transmission of thought, and without thought there would be no mankind.

I am not one of those pessimists who say that too much is being said and written in the medical world today. Quite the contrary, I believe that we should talk and write still more, but that we should do it better, and only when we have something positive to say, something that will stimulate, or inform, disclose or confirm some fact or finding that will be of value to other physicians.

The Problem of Medical Communication 69

It is useless to complain about the excessive number of medical works published everyday. The printed word is here to stay, and everyday it will increase in quantity.* Instead of mourning the fact that the physician cannot simplify his existence by bringing it down to a single medical text, like the physicians of Plato's Greece, and do without medical magazines, like the physicians up to 1679 when Nicholas de Blegny, surgeon to Louis XIV and his queen, founded the first medical journal, *Nouvelles Découvertes sur toutes les Parties de la Médicine,* let us accept the state of affairs as it is. Let us be glad that there is such a plethora of material on which to draw and set our wits to work to devise the best form in which to make proper use of it.

Ethical values in medicine, such as the relationship between physician and patient, are eternal and immutable. The idea that society has regarding the patient may change, as it changed, for instance, from the ancient Babylonian concept of him as a sinner to the primitive Christian concept of the patient as a potential saint. The basic principles of medicine, however, do not vary. The physician continues to be both an artist and a man of science, for he requires not only science and experience but also intuition and skill, just like any practitioner of an art. Let us not forget the common origin of art and medicine. To the ancient Greeks medicine was *techne* (craft) and the physician was a craftsman, like the sculptor or carpenter, and in Leonardo's Florence, painters were members of the Guild of Physicians and Apothecaries, through whose good offices they purchased their pigments.

As a man of science, the physician must communicate his discoveries so that others may benefit from them and that they may remain on record. As an artist, he must also do so if he is to exercise his profession efficiently and with skill. When the physician imparts something he has learned because he wishes to make a contribution to scientific progress, he is helping medicine *as a science;* when he does it because he wishes to assist others with his empirical knowledge, he is helping medicine *as an art.*

THE TRANSIENT NATURE OF MEDICAL PAPERS

Unfortunately medical documents enjoy but a short life. This is a point worthy of our consideration. A work of art is immortal. The frescoes and murals that thrilled the residents of imperial Pompeii stir our emotions to this day. That "Moses" by Michelangelo in front of which the Doges stood in ecstasy in the church of San Pietro de

---

* There are more than 10,000 medical journals in the world, and more than 3000 books on medicine are published every year.

Vincoli in Rome had the same effect on Sigmund Freud four hundred years later. And while the world lasts, the sculptures of Phidias, the canvases of El Greco, the Taj Mahal, the massive granite of the Escorial, and the exquisite chased chalices of Benvenuto Cellini will continue to fill the soul of man with wonder.

A medical paper, however, has a very short life. Apart from the Hippocratic Collection, the Treatises of Galen, and the Canon of Avicenna, that sacred trilogy which universally held first place for more than fifteen centuries, we need take only one glance through Boerhaave's "Pathology," which was a lamp of learning for the whole of Europe during the seventeenth century, Kraepelin's "Psychiatry" in the last century, or even the latest "Endocrinology" by Falta, to perceive that apart from their historical value none of them has withstood the passage of time and medical progress.

Furthermore, the span of life, the life expectation of a medical document becomes shorter every passing day as we continue our advances in medical science. The descriptions of pneumonia, typhoid and other infectious diseases in Osler's original textbook have succumbed to the impact of antibiotics as far as their natural history is concerned. The natural history and biologic cycles of disease will change as and when new drugs are discovered.

To cite a current example, the picture of mental diseases will vary as much in the next ten years with the use of ataraxics as that of infections has varied during the last fifteen years with the use of antibiotics. All this will only aggravate the problem of medical communication by demanding that each and every record be constantly rectified and brought up to date as further progress is made. Hence the pressing need to increase the flow and rhythm of medical communication. In another paper[1] I explained some of the problems of medical communication as follows:

> The greatest problem of modern medicine is that of communication: communication not only between the physician and the sick person, so indispensable particularly in psychiatry, but also between the investigator and his problems, the clinician and the patient, and the educator and his pupils. Especially vital is the need to communicate scientific finding, clinical data, medical discoveries, or the great-in-its-humbleness daily medical experience to the professional who needs to know all this in order to fulfill better his ministry. Despite the progress in radio, films, and television, books and journals are still the best vehicles of medical communication.
>
> "There are only three pleasures in life pure and lasting and all derived from inanimate things—books, pictures and the face of nature," said William Hazlitt. These three supreme components are represented in a medical journal by the word, the image, and the phenomena of human nature whether normal or suffering from that painful "mode of life" that we call disease.

The Problem of Medical Communication

"In the beginning was the Word . . ." and in the beginning as well as in the end the written word and the image were and will be the most faithful messenger of medical thought.

In the world of medicine, events occur in the hospital ward, in the physician's office, or in the research laboratory. After these phenomena have been recorded by the eyes and ears of the observers or by the camera's magic pupil, they are transmuted into words and images that later, on the printing presses, are converted through electrical impulses and mechanical vibrations into articles and photographs which, lastly, are integrated into the pages of a medical journal. As happens in every biologic cycle, this process is a continuing one. Readers of medical journals transmute in their minds the words and images into ideas and concepts that will help them in carrying on their research, clinical practice, or medical teaching, thus creating new links in this endless chain of development.

Medical journals integrate the three categories established by Osler —"creators, transmuters and transmitters"—since they create a climate of opinion around scientific problems, transmute phenomena and events into ideas and concepts, and transmit to their readers not only the golden stream of classical medical wisdom, but also that other "small" daily clinical wisdom which, like a fine rain of gold dust, is daily precipitated upon the mind of the general practitioner.

What can be done to solve the problems of medical communication in the case we are concerned with—in the field of antibiotic medicine?

THE BASIC PROBLEM OF MEDICAL COMMUNICATION

First of all, what are the basic problems of medical communication? In my opinion there are four: (1) To ensure that every valuable medical or scientific discovery, theoretical or practical, shall be published, and as soon as possible, cutting down to the minimum the period elapsing between the moment of discovery and that of its communication to the rest of the profession; (2) to ensure a world-wide distribution for every medical text to any physician who needs it, overcoming geographic and language barriers; (3) to organize, coordinate, and integrate all antibiotic knowledge into an efficient and always up-to-the-minute source of antibiotic data; and (4) to guarantee maximum speed in incorporating into medical practice any reported scientific advance by translating it into adequate practical measures.

Such a program of ideal objectives in the field of medical communication would help to bring about a revolution in service to the physician and consequently to the sick, who are dependent upon how much and how soon the physician learns of the newest advances in medicine.

Medicine is becoming more technical and more specialized everyday. This the general practitioner feels more than anyone else, for everyday it becomes more difficult for him to obtain and master such knowledge and integrate into his own practice the most important advances in each particular specialty. Although specialization existed in previous historical periods, medical learning in those times was not extensive enough to create problems for the general practitioner, as it does today.

What, then, can we do to solve these problems?

First, we should recognize one principle that is often utterly disregarded: the most important thing in medicine is *not* to report one's findings; the most important thing in medicine is *to communicate, to propagate one's findings.*

No one, as far as I know, has ever stressed this most basic principle. There is a world of difference between "reporting" and "communicating." The Spaniard Servet "reported" his discovery of pulmonary circulation in his treatise "Restitutio Christianismi," published in 1553; but it was not until many years later that his discovery was fully "communicated" and accepted by the medical world. The same thing occurred with the discovery of percussion by Auenbrugger, vaccination by Jenner, x-rays by Roentgen, and antiseptic surgery by Lister. Two Austrian investigators, Meyer and Nally, reported the synthesis of isoniazid in an obscure paper published in the journal, *Monatshefte der Chemie,* but it was not until 1952 that it was made known to the medical world and tested in pulmonary tuberculosis. Fleming dutifully reported his discovery of penicillin in 1928; but it was not until 1940 that, thanks to Florey and Chain, his discovery was placed at the service of mankind.

History abounds with cases of important discoveries buried among the dusty pages of some unknown publication that not until many years later were wrested from oblivion, studied, and applied. Today this happens far too often, with the result that several scientists may be duplicating each other's work, or that one man may devote his life to repeating work already carried out by someone else many years before, or that thousands of physicians the world over may be deprived of the benefit of a multitude of scientific advances that would make their work easier and more efficient. *Much is reported but not enough is communicated.* Reports are minute editorial pebbles cast on the waters of the wide lake of medical literature, whose expanding ripples die out before they reach those on the distant banks who could put them to proper use.

ON THE ART OF CLEAR WRITING

What can be done to remedy this state of affairs?

Above all, the physician must report and impart everything that may be of theoretical or practical value to others. It is not enough to know something for oneself; it must be imparted to everyone else. The distinction is the same as that existing between a poor instructor who imparts but a fraction of his knowledge and a true teacher who teaches everything he knows.

The mere fact of expressing in words a discovery of any kind is already a means to making it permanent, to understanding it and improving it further. The written word is the most dynamic force on earth. Harvey's winged words started the medical revolution that led to present-day physiology; Fleming's simple description of his discovery initiated the antibiotic revolution; Freud's bold words changed the whole field of medical anthropology and psychopathology. Too many physicians and research workers are afraid to reveal their findings, because, for example, they may be based on one single case or on a small group of cases, or because the data obtained are negative.

Referring only to these two reasons for silence, I would stress that the single case in medicine, just like the single and isolated earthquake or flood in geology, may be of the greatest instructional value, while a negative result may well be the key that opens the door to a whole treasurehouse of positive results. It is therefore imperative to write and communicate everything you know, distilling into written words the unique and valuable experience of every individual.

Writing and publishing one's knowledge may be stimulated by closer contact between the author and the editors of medical journals, which are the most universal means of medical communication. The mission of the public censor is to say, "You can't do that!"; but the editor's job is to say, "That's the way to do it!" The editor works constantly in the field of medical communication, and his advice, inspiration, and guidance may be invaluable to many physicians and research workers less expert in this art.

I believe that no fixed rules can be laid down for the writing of good medical literature. This may smack a little of heresy, coming as it does from one who has devoted a good part of his life to medical communication. Nevertheless, I repeat, I do not believe in fixed rules for writing good medical literature. Suppose there had been applied to the writings of Osler, Oliver Wendell Holmes, Cajal, Mackenzie, and Freud those strict rules that some people now recommend—the methodically clipped phrase, short, simple words, avoidance of all rare, rich, or colorful expressions—then medical literature would have been deprived of some of its greatest masterworks. I do believe, however, that there are certain principles of good writing whether it be on medicine, art, mathematics, carpentry, or travel. The principles of "lucidity, simplicity, and euphony" recommended to young writers by Somerset Maugham in "The Summing Up" are indeed the best rules one can think of for the creation of good literature in the medical world also. Literature is an invaluable aid to medicine. Did not Thomas Sydenham advise Blackmore to learn medicine by reading *Don Quixote*?

SYMBOLS, METAPHORS, AND THE SEMANTIC PROBLEM

We must withal improve our art of communication by learning to write more and better, so as to arrive at some common denominator in medicine that may smooth the path for physicians and investigators throughout the world to understand one another better. This brings us to the point of the problem of semantics in medical communication.

Man's greatest invention has been signs and symbols, i.e., written signs or sounds representing objects and ideas. From the moment he is born, man has to face all sorts of problems and situations. To solve these, man uses signs and symbols as a means of recalling past problems, cataloguing his present ones, and anticipating those of the future. In turn, he applies to such symbols the principles and rules derived from what we call science, grammar, logic, or physics.

Symbols, however, are not always accurate or trustworthy. Every human being has his own inner picture of the external world, a picture that differs with every person, since it is formed exclusively by what each one personally knows or imagines about things, people, and places in the outer world. In his turn, each person reflects and projects upon the world and upon all other creatures his inner picture of the world, partial and inexact though it perforce always is. It is as though the world were reflected in millions of mirrors—the individual minds of man—every one of them with a different radius of curvature; all reflections therefore are different.

If we bear this in mind, the problem of human communication becomes simplified when everyone recognizes that his picture of the world and of things is not the only one, that it is no more accurate than anybody else's, and, above all, that *it is only an image* and not the external, objective reality. If we make a thousand people walk by a painting, or if we read them a poem, or show them a film, or play a sonata for them, each person will have an impression different from that of the others. The mission of science is necessarily to restore the true value and meaning of our symbols, remembering all the time that they are only metaphors for reality and not immutable dogma. That is the way science attains its greatest dignity and efficiency. For, while dogma has been the historic ballast to theology, metaphor has been the flying wing of science.

The secret of progress in medical communication therefore depends on accepting that symbols shall represent not individual images, not the engrams within each human mind, but objects and facts that are objective expressions of the interrelationships between things, creatures, and realities in the outside world. Precision and objectiveness in scientific language and proper use of symbols as representations of external correlations are an indispensable condition for satisfactory communication between men in the field of medical science.

A NEW CONCEPT OF MEDICAL JOURNALISM

Where must we publish? Wherever we can, but we should try to reach those journals that have a receptive intellectual audience.

I firmly believe in the social and scientific mission of the medical publications distributed free to physicians, so much so that I am already connected with a journal that is sent free to a great number of physicians without its ethical and professional character being jeopardized. In this manner, I feel, we are anticipating the future. For the physician of tomorrow will have *free* access to many publications for which he at present has to pay and to which he is often unable to subscribe.

The mission of a medical publication is *to communicate,* and if the only way to fulfill this mission is to send it gratis to the profession, then by all means let us take this bold yet constructive step forward in the art of medical communication. The proof that such a step is only anticipating by a few years the medical world of tomorrow, when physicians will receive free most of the professional publications to which they now have to subscribe, is that the great pharmaceutical companies that have been revolutionary pioneers in the field of antibiotic medicine have already recognized this need. Their assistance to scientific publications, by means of their advertisements, is helping to solve that vital problem of medical communication; to bring out at the *earliest* possible date, to as *many* people as possible, the *greatest number* of the *best* possible medical works. In another paper,[2] where I discussed the present and future of medical advertising, I stated the following:

> The third important source of scientific information for the physician today, a source worthy of a place alongside textbooks and medical journals, is the scientific literature prepared and sent to physicians by pharmaceutical companies.
> Only a few years ago such literature was considered—rightfully so—mere advertising propaganda, in the worst sense of the term. Today the medical literature issued by pharmaceutical companies, and

often prepared by medical advertising agencies, has become an important source of study, consultation, reference, and medical education. Specifically in the fields of antibiotics, vitamins, biological products, and hormones, it can be said that pharmaceutical literature is not only abundant but also precise, effective, ethical, and educational.

To a certain degree, the evolution of pharmaceutical advertising has followed a course which I would compare to the evolution of painting in history. Classical painting represented especially the physical bulk of objects and persons; the impressionists relegated photographic representation of physical bulk to a subordinate level and presented lights and shadows; modern surrealistic art represents the idea of things, the very soul of an object. For Velázquez, a human being was the specular image of his physical make-up; for Seurat, the human being was a conglomerate of tiny dots of polychrome light; for Picasso, he is a geometric abstraction. Summing up, classical art represents *things;* impressionism, the *light* of things; modern art, the *idea* of things. Classical art is photographic and visual; impressionism appeals to the sensory and emotional image; modern art, to the intelligence as it presents *the concept* of things.

Pharmaceutical advertising began by presenting a photograph of the *products* followed by a verbal description and a cumbersome iconography. All past pharmaceutical literature is cluttered with bottles, pills, ampules, and salve tubes. The revolution began when such advertising represented *the properties* and uses of the products involved. Modern pharmaceutical literature presents *the idea* behind a given product, the philosophic concept that motivates and justifies it. A recent campaign of pharmaceutical advertising on the combined use of antibiotics and vitamins for treating the etiologic agent of an infection and the stress caused by it was successfully based on the introduction of such a concept into medical thought and later on the introduction of the product incarnating that idea.

In my opinion, the medical literature of the future—including medical advertising—will shed its present form and become *educational literature*. When a drug is universally accepted and becomes a part of the basic therapeutic arsenal of the physician, it no longer needs any advertising: it is enough to inform, guide, and educate us in how to use it. A vaccine, a hormone, an antibiotic already tried and proved does not need advertising; all we need is technical information on how to use it. As I see it, medicopharmaceutical advertising in the future will be limited to announcing new products, while its primary mission will be educational to complete the work of preventive medicine which is the Medicine of the Future.

Meanwhile, for a physician who can winnow the wheat from the praises heaped on, let us say, a drug; one who has an eye for picking the nuggets out of a mine of information; for him pharmaceutical literature is a precious source of medical knowledge and an educational vehicle of unique value. This is especially true of physicians who practice in remote regions where it takes months for a book or a journal to arrive. This "country doctor" keeps abreast of the progress of medicine through a flood of pamphlets, leaflets, and advertisements as colorful as a peacock's plumes but containing information as scientific and precise as the calculations done by a Princeton mathematician.

A medical publication should not be an ivory tower; it should be an open forum accessible to all physicians and research workers where they may speak freely to all their colleagues. In theory as in practice, that is what I think, and that is the way I have directed the course of our modest contribution to the solution of the problem of medical communication in the field of antibiotics.

CHAIRS IN ANTIBIOTIC MEDICINE AND THE INTERNATIONAL ANTIBIOTIC INSTITUTE

But what can one or even several publications do? A great deal more must be done and that on an international scale. Herman T. Biggs once made a statement that became the motto of the New York State Public Health Department: *"Public health is purchasable; within natural limitations any community can determine its own death rate."* So also might we say that medical communication can be financed, and within certain limits each medical community can determine the degree of knowledge its members may attain.

Who better than the pharmaceutical industry could organize, coordinate, and integrate on an international scale the vast and increasing knowledge on antibiotics?

From this platform in past years I have launched my call, which I now repeat, to the pharmaceutical industry to establish Chairs in Antibiotic Medicine in various countries of the world and to set up an International Institute of Antibiotics dedicated exclusively to organizing knowledge in this field, a center to act as a universal brain for receiving, classifying, synthesizing, and making available all printed material on antibiotics. Such an international center, by means of its publications, chairs, traveling professors, iconographies, and museums, could solve the problem of world-wide communication of antibiotic knowledge, which in turn would ensure increasing progress in antibiotic medicine.

This is no castle in Spain, no Utopian vision; it is an all-compelling necessity that will aid both the abstract science and the practical art of medicine. Such an institution might very well help the modern physician to become what two thousand years ago that magnificent Athenian, Plato, demanded: the medical statesman—the *Asklepios politikos.*

WORDS AND RESEARCH

For the fifth time in as many years, physicians, investigators, and clinicians of many nationalities are gathered here to cement further the bonds of friendship, to assess the year's harvest in antibiotics, and to gaze at the new day rising above the historical horizon.

MAN AND HIS PROBLEMS

The object of this Symposium is easy to define. Like that other famous symposium recorded by Plato and presided over by the physician Eryximachus amidst the quiet silver-green shades of the Greek countryside, we have gathered here to discuss problems of mutual interest. That we *have* problems indicates that, more than scientists, we are human beings, for only man has problems. It is the very fact of his problems, wherefrom spring all his misery and all his greatness, that makes man human.

The dictionary defines the world "problem" as a "question proposed for solution." Etymologically the word derives from the Greek *pro* and *blepo,* meaning something thrown before our eyes. Any difficulty one may encounter—physical, economic, intellectual, or, as in our case, scientific—is therefore a problem.[1]

Our problem is to develop fresh weapons for combating diseases in general and infectious diseases in particular. This is a scientific problem. We must also render these weapons into instruments that will

---

Delivered at the Fifth Annual Symposium on Antibiotics, Washington, D. C., October 2–4, 1957.

help us understand the natural history of a disease and the biologic cycle of its causal germs. This is a historical problem, for it affects the knowledge and advances of our time.

To each one of us individually, scientific research involves at least one of the two afore-mentioned problems. Were this not so we would not be here at this meeting. Whatever our particular interest may be —clinical, experimental, biochemical, industrial, agricultural, veterinarian, or, as in my case, historical—research to all of us philosophically represents something vital. This is so much so, that we have traveled here only to tell one another what we have thought and done and what we contemplate doing further in the antibiotic field. Reporting our thoughts and our past or future work is, in short, the intrinsic purpose of this Symposium.

WORDS AND MEDICINE

Were we to ask a historian living at the turn of our present millennium exactly what did, say, 800 people, which is our number here today, do year after year at symposiums, I am sure he would answer, "Talk." But to talk is to use words to communicate. Nothing, then, is more fitting than to spend a few minutes together speaking about words as a means of communication.

Words, whether spoken or written, are the most powerful means of communication between human beings. From the time when the last Neolithic men developed a speech system until the invention several centuries later of tablet writing in Assyria and papyrus writing in Egypt, speech was the sole means of communicating and transmitting knowledge. Until the printing press was invented in the fifteenth century, the spoken word was the paramount vehicle for medical instruction, and ours indeed was the most *vocal* of all professions. Then, when human knowledge began to be transmitted in print, there came a reversion of medical pathology to its original *visual* form.

Nowadays the written word, after a transient period of domination over the spoken word, has to wage incessant battle against our modern radio, television, and electronic methods of transmitting voices and sounds, which now seem to be the predominant and most powerful means of communication between men. For all that, the written word may yet come out the winner. In the antibiotic field, the volume of scientific information published in the last 15 years is far greater than that in any other field of contemporary medicine.

WORDS AND TECHNOLOGY

Some of you may possibly be asking yourselves why are we devoting so much attention to words in a Symposium whose foremost objective is medical technology—that is, the practical application of scientific knowledge to the solution of problems of direct practical importance. The answer is that words form the most important facet of human personality and particularly of the scientist's personality, for science is based on the transmission and assimilation of knowledge.

Anatomists and philosophers have not, even yet, agreed on a definition of what Man is. However, we do know—as Singer[2] has pointed out—that all men possess one characteristic in common that distinguishes them from all other creatures—man makes things. But then, so do certain animals. Man fashions tools and instruments out of various objects, but so do a few animals. But only man can make tools with which to make still other tools! The most characteristic and constructive—and sometimes the most destructive—of all the instruments fashioned by man are *words*.

Animals use actions and sounds as *signals;* only man learned to use them as *symbols*. This was the simplest form of technologic advance. Man became proficient as a toolmaker and tool-user simply because he was a *maker* and *user* of words. Only after making considerable progress in constructing language, that is, in the technology of creating symbols, did he acquire the ability to improve his tools. Ever since then, for half a million years now, man has been making words and tools.*

WORDS AND MEDICAL PATHOLOGY

I am a physician and a historian speaking to persons with a vested interest in the diseased. Hence, I am in a position to maintain that medical progress throughout the ages has always been founded upon fresh methods of "looking at" the morbid reality that is the patient. Hippocrates looked at the patient as a sufferer; Galen viewed him as a function not only of his humors but also of his diseased organs,

---

* It took man hundreds of thousands of years before he ceased to rely on his hands alone in collecting food, and became a hunter and fisherman with arrowheads and spears made of flint and stone, bone and wood. Two facts in this pageant of history are worthy of note: first, for a million years mankind made little or no progress in using his hands, then reached the highest skill in the days of ancient Egypt and Babylon; and second, technologic proficiency in the Far East was always far ahead of anything in Western Europe. While Greek thinkers were weaving philosophies more tenuous than the finest gossamer, the Chinese had already invented gunpowder, block printing, projectiles, ceramics, cosmetics and plastic surgery, anesthesia, and even the pocket handkerchief; meanwhile Plato and Aristotle were still wiping their honorable and learned noses on the inside of their togas.

Words and Research   81

much as we ourselves do these days; Morgagni related the patient's symptoms to determinate internal organs, which in turn inspired Laënnec's work; Addison, with his investigations of the suprarenal cortex, showed that endocrine lesions were possibly the core of certain diseases; Claude Bernard—that mighty figure who was not a physiologist but Physiology itself in human form—taught us to think physiologically, to base our opinions not only on experimental data and statistics but also on the normalities and abnormalities of the body processes; Virchow brought this notion down to the level of the cell; Pasteur initiated the "tyranny" of the microbe, which was to last so many years; and Ehrlich and Fleming contributed not only fresh forms of therapy but also fresh approaches to the problem of disease, fresh vantage points from which to track down the sources of disease. But all these men, with the exception of Galen, had one factor in common: They were able *lucidly* and *accurately* to report their observations of the sick human being.

An example of how lucidity in reporting may affect the results thereof is provided by the interesting fact, revealed by Arthur Jores, Professor of Medical Pathology at Hamburg, and commented on by Rof Carballo,[3] that of the 2000 human diseases recorded in textbooks the etiology of not more than 800 is known. Of the many of the rest—asthma, gastric ulcer, hypertension, for instance—we know in detail many of their pathogenic peculiarities, but we know little about their true etiology.

These diseases, whose pathogenesis is known and whose etiology remains unknown, are diseases specific to mankind; they are not observed in identical fashion among animals. On the other hand, those diseases against which we have efficient etiologic countermeasures are the ones man has in common with the higher mammals. Present-day pathology is "prosthetic," not etiologic, for it makes only temporary, prosthetic replacements; it is etiologic only in so far as it relates to the pathology of the higher mammals.*

Progress has been greater in those fields—such as the naturalistic description of human and mammal pathology—in which reporting has been clearer and more precise and hence less theoretic or interpretive.

Infectious diseases are an excellent example of how accuracy and excellence of description, from Hippocrates to our own time, can smooth the path of research. On the other hand, in schizophrenia, atherosclerosis, asthma, and cancer, multiplicity of interpretation and semantic confusion have greatly hindered diagnosis and therapy. The

---

* Thomas Sydenham already stated that acute diseases were *biologic* or *animal* (or, as we say today, epidemiologic) and that chronic diseases were *biographic* or *human* (or, in our language, psychosomatic or degenerative).

better we learn how to describe the etiology, symptoms, and course of a disease, the easier it will be to hit upon the proper treatment.

Clear, detailed, and prompt reporting is therefore an active, vital part of the solution to medical problems.

WORDS, SEARCH, AND RESEARCH

Two prior steps are involved before an investigator undertakes the task of making a report in actual words. In the first place, he must have *thought* about a particular problem, that is, it must have preoccupied him; second, he must have *done* something about it, that is, he must have occupied himself in investigating that problem. Only after such meditative and cognitive acts will he perform the conative act of communicating his thoughts and experiments in the form of a scientific paper.

Inquiring thought, probably the oldest thinking in medicine, began when man started to explore the world and discovered how to use fire, metals, the ax, wheel, and lever, and how to make pottery. During succeeding ages it bloomed into the analytic thinking of the Greek philosophers and the introduction of the first experiments capable of reproduction. In this path of progress, alongside the work of the Italian scientific academies and the Invisible College in London, which replaced the medieval universities, men like Galileo, Harvey, Newton, and Haller stand out brilliantly. Their curiosity and self-abnegation gave new life to the noble Aristotelian tradition of wanting to know the reason for things and to understand Nature scientifically.

In every investigation the *search* for elementary data, often of a morphologic character, preceded the search for the dynamic interrelationships amongst objects, i.e., *research* properly so-called. The flame has always preceded the light. So also the thirst for learning is born with human life. Aren't children always asking the how, what, and why of things? The eyes of the researcher light up with the same curiosity as a child's eyes, which look at everything in astonishment and wonder.

The scientific investigator who, as Cicero counseled, "strives to render himself strange to the familiar," converts such curiosity into a guide in his work. In finding his way through the jungle of fact, the investigator must be guided by his imagination as a navigator is guided by the distant stars. Imagination can be a torch to illuminate his path, but he must always be ready to recognize that, as Huxley said, "the tragedy of all inquiry is that a beautiful hypothesis may be slain by an ugly fact." He must allow that not every experiment ends in achievement, and he must appreciate the value of negative data.

If, besides, he admits that his research is founded upon the work of his predecessors and feels himself at one with them in time and space, his investigation will then become the mission, direction, and glory of his life.

The inquiring mind has altered little in its basic directives throughout human history. Hildebrand[4] brilliantly describes how Merezhkovski wrote in *The Romance of Leonardo da Vinci* of a "duel of learning" that took place in the court of Duke Ludovico il Moro in Milan in the year 1498. There were gathered "sundry doctors, deans, and magisters of the University of Pavia, in quadrangular red caps, in scarlet silk capes, lined with ermine, in gloves of violet chamois, with gold-embroidered pouches at their belts. The ladies of the court were in gorgeous ball apparel.

"Soon the Countess Cecilia proposed to the Duke that he ask Leonardo to take part in the tourney. His topic was sea shells.

"His exposition was received with hostility. An old doctor of scholastics maintained that 'the disputation was being carried on improperly,' because 'either the problem . . . belonged to the lower, "mechanical" knowledge, foreign to metaphysics, in which case there was nothing to be said of it, inasmuch as they had not convened here to contend over subjects not related to philosophy, or else the problem was related to the true, higher knowledge—to dialectics; in such case, it must even be discussed in accordance with the laws of dialectics, raising the subjects to pure mental contemplation.'

" 'There is no higher or lower knowledge,' Leonardo replied, 'but one only, flowing out of experimentation. . . . For, in considering subjects not open to proof, men cannot come to any agreement. Where there are no sensible deductions, their place is taken by shouts. But he that knoweth hath no need of shouting.'

"Upon this, bedlam broke loose, but Leonardo was silent. He perceived his isolation among these people, . . . saw the uncrossable abyss that separated them from him."

But that thought of Leonardo's still inspires science today and the methodology of research.*

INDUSTRY AND RESEARCH

Research methodology has been put to its best use by industry,

---

* This methodology might be summarized in four stages: (1) fortuitous or deliberate observation of an incident; (2) immediate provisional hypothesis; (3) search for significant data to confirm or refute the original hypothesis; (4) new hypothesis, tested by observation and experimentation.

Such methodology is founded on the force of ideas, since, as Claude Bernard taught, "the idea is the seed, the method the soil in which it flourishes. Since only what is sown will grow, nothing will develop by the experimental method except *the ideas* submitted to it."

MEN, MOLDS, AND HISTORY

which these days is giving tremendous aid to the researcher, particularly in the antibiotic field. Research itself has become an industry in its own right, for by creating new products and opening up fresh markets it has added a dynamic strength to world economy. Industries no longer compete in markets but in the creation of new necessities, so as to determine what discoveries need to be made and then make them. Industry has found that it is possible to harness science and invention with production, to systematize the search for knowledge, and, by having huge research teams working simultaneously on the same project, to achieve in a few months what otherwise would take years or even decades.

ART, MEDICINE, AND SCIENCES

Equally important in understanding the language of science are the interrelationships between art, medicine, and other sciences.

In what we today call "Modern" art, despite the fact that Gauguin, van Gogh, and Cézanne all painted their pictures before the turn of the century, the influence of scientific progress has been enormous—as Melicow[5] has pointed out—not because the artists themselves were well versed in science, but because the cultural atmosphere of their day was so permeated with it that it could not but influence their minds and, consequently, their work. Thus, the discovery of the refraction of white light through a prism into the colors of the spectrum had its artistic reflex in Seurat's *pointillism,* the splitting of light into an infinite number of separate, luminous dots of color on canvas; the new notions on physics and on form and light illuminated *impressionism,* the rendering with the brush subjective impressions of outer reality, as in the paintings of Manet, Monet, and Pissarro; the explorations into the unconscious were related to *expressionism,* or the projection of the painter's mind and feelings onto his work, as in the case of van Gogh; fragmentation of the human frame and penetration into its inmost tissues and recesses consequent to the discovery of roentgen rays and the progress of radiology influenced the original *cubism* of Braque and Picasso; atom-splitting physics with its threat of universal disintegration was reflected in the works of abstract painters and in Dali's atomic fragmentation; the modern concept of the unity of time and space forming a single space-time continuum is evident in Picasso's later work, which depicts one and the same person, both full-face and profile, at various ages on the same canvas, together with views of his body seen from different angles, thus introducing a new *time* dimension into painting—a hitherto purely *spatial* art. Lastly, the advances since Freud in psychiatry and psychology illuminated Kandinsky's *nonobjective* art and the *surrealism* of Miró, Tanguy, Klee, and de Chirico.

Words and Research

In present-day scientific research, such integration of thought has ousted the fragmentation of scientific findings. Thus, the electrical industry has provided us with new chemical substances; modern mathematics has aided neurologists in charting of brain maps; the hydraulic pumps of the automobile industry have been modified and used in hospitals to pump liquefied foods into the stomachs of patients just operated upon, thereby sometimes eliminating the need for intravenous feeding; and another improvement in the same industry, a sensitive apparatus for testing car parts, has been employed in the development of an electronic stethoscope.

THE DUTY OF BEING LUCID

The harvest of the investigation that constitutes the second step in research is finally put into words. These words must be transparently clear. Lucidity of expression is synonymous with quality of thought. The more of a naturalist a scientist is, that is, the more he observes natural phenomena and the less he theorizes, the clearer his thinking becomes.

The lack of progress in psychiatry during the past 50 years, barring Freud's contributions to medical anthropology, may well be attributed to the fact that, although psychiatry deals with the obstacles that forfeit man's ability to communicate with his fellow men, it has failed to express itself clearly. For half a century psychiatry has employed a strange language ever more and more confusing and obscure. Fortunately, it is now pulling itself out of this mire, thanks to the success of physiodynamic and organicist psychiatry, which speaks the plain, clear language of biology. Thanks to this, numerous successes have been achieved during the last five years in the psychochemotherapeutic field, and many more will no doubt follow these, until one day the sphinx of mental disease will finally surrender its secret.

This goal demands that psychiatrists cease to be mystics and theoreticians and become biologists and physicians in their explorations into the tenebrous world of mental disease.

THE WORD, CREATOR OF KNOWLEDGE

Antibiotic medicine, on the other hand, has progressed considerably in a few years because it has used a clear, definite, biologic language. In chemistry, biochemistry, pharmacology, and clinical medicine, only one vocabulary is possible, that of biologic science. In biology each term has a unique meaning. Lack of lucidity occurs mostly when we formulate new concepts. Now, without new concepts to integrate the results of research, no progress can be made. Hence, it is indispensable that the scientist convey his thoughts with lucidity, clothing them as tights clothe the circus acrobat, without hiding their form.

It is also essential for the researcher to learn that, whatever his field, he must complement the study of things in *space* (which is the function of *science*) with the study of events in *time* (which is the mission of *history*) and with the study of the basic concepts of life in its biologic, social, universal, and human aspects (which is *philosophy*).

A lucid philosophy of science has led to our present advances. That is why the fabric of the scientist's words, if these are to become his basic instrument in expressing his thoughts, must be woven from his combined knowledge of science, history, and philosophy. This does not mean that he must become a bookworm and forsake his scientific chores for the theoretical study of these other subjects. It does mean, however, that at all times he ought to know how to keep a total perspective, seeing things, as Spinoza says, *sub specie aeternitatis* (in view of eternity) and *sub specie totius* (in view of totality).*

To live perceptively in this manner—as an investigator, as a man with a sense of history, who bears in mind that our present work is the result of the heritage handed us by our forebears and itself the heritage of the future, and as a philosopher at heart who loves wisdom although he never attains it, just as sailors never reach the stars they follow on their path across the ocean—to live thus is to be a complete man. He who is able to do this will always speak with the clear, simple, friendly tongue of the biologist and the naturalist.

THE WORD, CREATOR OF HUMANITY

Words, however, have another mission besides imparting knowledge—a most important mission in a Symposium such as this, where old friends meet year after year and where they become acquainted with new friends as well. That mission is for us to approach each other and, by talking among ourselves, to turn our cosmic loneliness into companionship. It is, perhaps, the noblest work that words can do—to act as carriers of sincere friendship among men. For the simple act of two people meeting and stirring the air with the sound of words of greeting establishes the human bases of history with all its glory and grandeur.

---

* The investigator must do that with the same *tenacity, humility,* and *passion* that Pavlov recommended as the three greatest attributes of the inquiring mind. He must not seek to possess the truth but to become a philosopher in the true original meaning of the word, namely, a "lover of wisdom," a lover fated—as in Keats's "Ode on a Grecian Urn"—never to possess but always to desire and adore, for it is far more rewarding to wish than to possess.

THE MEANING OF GREATNESS

SIR ALEXANDER FLEMING—IN MEMORIAM

Greatness is simplicity. "To be great," said Nietzsche, "is to point out new directions. . . ."—We might add, to point them out with elegant simplicity. The death of Sir Alexander Fleming, a great man of great simplicity, invites us to ponder once again the meaning of greatness. It is sad but inevitable that no sooner are the great scientific conceptions of the human mind incorporated into man's treasure store of wisdom than they eclipse their creators. Artistic creation, on the other hand, is linked inextricably with the personality of the creator. One cannot hear the chords of *Eroica* without recalling the pensive, leonine head of Beethoven; one cannot read a page of *Don Quixote* without thinking of the man who penned it; one cannot gaze upon the *Night Watch* without seeing the melancholy figure of Rembrandt.

But this is not true of scientific creation. As it grows it becomes more and more impersonal, until finally it detaches itself completely from the person of its creator. How many people inoculated with smallpox vaccine know the name of Jenner? How many tubercular patients could identify Koch? How many luetics have given a thought to Ehrlich? Scientific achievements, unlike artistic achievements, do not endure in terms of their originators; the scientist himself feels subconsciously that his glory is transitory, that his name will vanish as soon as the formula, the medicine, or the heavenly body he discovered passes into common domain. The more concrete are the outlines of his work, the more indistinct does his personality, and even his name, become in the mists of time.

But in the history of modern medicine, Fleming is the one scientist whose name and personality are most often recognized in connection with his scientific accomplishments. One day I was having luncheon with Sir Alexander and Lady Fleming in Rome. On the table, fragrant fruits were piled high in golden wicker baskets garnished with fresh greens. Sir Alexander had just returned from my native Spain and his eyes were still aglow with the heavenly lights of Andalusia. Everywhere in the dusty villages people had kissed his hand as they would that of a saint; even the gypsies milled around his car on the dusty roads to Granada to catch a glimpse of him. In Athens he attended a performance of *Medea*. When he went backstage to compliment the star, she fell on her knees and, tears misting her eyes, she said: "If it had not been for *your* penicillin, I would not be alive to perform in this theatre today."

Fleming became in his lifetime what few scientists ever become: a universal symbol of wisdom and goodness, a symbol of that "science which, had it no conscience, would be nothing but baseness of soul," as Montaigne, that jeweler of philosophic verities, once said. People perhaps sensed in this frail man, with limpid blue eyes, silvery white hair, and cheeks as rosy as the dawn over the Scottish moors, the mystic presence of an apostle of science.

Perhaps the reason Fleming's popularity transcended the limits of his achievements is that from the very beginning he was concerned with the *practical* application of penicillin. In 1928 a "fortunate accident" befell Fleming, as it has to many other scientists not nearly so well prepared to convert the firefly of a chance discovery into a new star. Fleming once said: "Don't wait for Fortune to smile on you. Prepare yourself with knowledge. Then, if Fortune presents an opportunity you will be able to take advantage of it." Yet ten years were to elapse before another scientist, Raistrick, reinvestigated penicillin, and two more years passed before other scientists, Florey and Chain, made practical clinical testing possible. The world rang with hope as it learned of the discovery that promised to liberate man from the cruelest scourge in history: infection. The scientist who thus ushered in a new era in medicine had wedded scientific observation to genius when he translated the vision of a laboratory investigator into a clinical reality.

Fleming's greatness was apparent from the very beginning in the simplicity of his person and of his conduct, which accentuated all the more the magnitude of his discovery. Our times are bountiful in *big* men—in industry, in finance, in politics—but they can boast of few *great* men. Fleming revealed himself to be a *great* man in whom the very frailty of his small frame and the softness of his voice contrasted with the simple but gigantic ideologic framework that supported the inner structure of his personality.

What manner of research scientist was Fleming? I would say he was a naturalist—an investigator of the Hippocratic school, enamored of the ancient aphorism *Medicina tota in observationibus,* capable of doing what Darwin advised: to contribute to man's knowledge of Nature, not so much by an ability to deliver theoretical disquisitions, as by knowing how to count dexterously and correctly the tiny leaves of a plant.

A truly good investigator is more of a naturalist than an experimenter. This can be said of Fleming. Medicine has always been and should always be, above all, a science based on empirical observation. The physician should learn not only to see, but to *look,* and he should then interpret correctly what he sees. Fleming discovered penicillin because of his training as a naturalist devoted to simple but consequential observation, the same training had by Pasteur, Lister, Hunter, and Claude Bernard, not to forget Cajal and Pavlov and other great naturalists in medicine.

The famous "accident" that befell Fleming, when some humble spores carried by smoky winds through the gray skies of London fell on his culture plate, had certainly occurred before in other laboratories. But it required a mind endowed with unique vision to perceive that such an accident was the gold-illuminated initial letter introducing a new and glorious chapter in the history of medicine. Fleming was guided by that "marvelous power of prolonged attention" recommended by Cajal.

Simplicity of thought, simplicity of feeling, simplicity in speech— all these gave meaning to Fleming's greatness. The form adopted by a scientific truth often becomes an integral part of the truth itself. Truth is, by definition, clear, and the art of expressing things clearly is of supreme importance in science. Scientific truth demands transparency, order, simplicity, precision, harmony. Hippocrates, Pasteur, Osler, and Freud fulfilled this demand. So did Alexander Fleming.

The clarity of his form, which contrasts with the rich significance of his prose—a limpid lake of calm but deep waters—is another of his claims to fame. Fleming's work is written in a plain, unadorned prose, comparable to that of Vergil's description of the swine plague in the *Georgics.* In Fleming's speeches and lectures, scientific thought was clad in a tunic of austere simplicity.

When a great man dies, the historical symbol is born. Antibiotics were introduced into modern medicine by Fleming's hand and were then transferred to the combined efforts of men in industry. As Fleming himself once said: "Who would have thought that a mold spore half the size of our blood corpuscles falling on one of my culture plates would eventually result in a large industry with factories employing thousands of people. . . ."

As time goes on, scientific work becomes more depersonalized, and it is finally remembered for its intrinsic value, not for the quality of the men who created it. But history bestowed upon Fleming the singular privilege of linking his name with his work as inextricably as Hamlet's words are associated with the genius of Shakespeare.

The Era of Antibiotics marches on with gigantic strides. Its progress is assured by complete depersonalization: the triumph of team work, complex instruments, well-appointed laboratories, and large-scale industries. But many years must pass before a patient treated with penicillin or the physician who administers it will forget the name of Fleming. This is the tribute to his greatness, infinitely more solemn than any wreath, that history has laid upon his tomb.

ON TREATING THE WHOLE PATIENT

Infection in man "mobilizes the entire organism in response to alarm warnings from those organic 'Pentagons' that comprise the pituitary-adrenal axis and the hypothalamic centers. . . ." [1] All the resources of the host are marshaled in an extended effort to overcome the invading microorganism.

Antibiotics, specific in their action, attack the etiologic agent involved in the infection without regard to other important requirements of the diseased tissue. Indeed, under certain conditions, antibiotics may even add to the patient's organic burden. Historically, antibiotic therapy represents the crystallization of the concept of frontal attack on the specific etiologic agents responsible for the various disease entities. This concept, originated by Pasteur during the nineteenth century, was further expanded by Koch and Lister, and finally fully developed by Ehrlich and Domagk in the last forty years. These men focused the treatment of disease on etiology as the best means of wiping out at one fell swoop the vast mural of symptoms and signs.

The objective of attacking the etiologic agent through chemicals attained its greatest expression with the advent of antibiotics. Modern medicine was then liberated from the empiricism of the last century, when the sick were "cured in textbooks" but "died in their beds." The physician neglected the "terrain," failing to realize that behind the microorganism and the consequent infection, there was a *sick man* whose normal nutritional requirements, because of tissue insults and a general condition of stress, were completely out of balance.

In the last century Bichat and Laënnec were champions of the anatomopathologic doctrine of disease, claiming that the basis of disease was the organic lesion. Other physiopathologists, like Claude Bernard, claimed that disease was a functional disorganization of the internal economy of the host; while a third group of etiopathologists, like Koch, believed that disease was merely an organic response to a specific etiologic agent. With Pasteur, Koch, Ehrlich, and later Fleming and other antibiotic investigators, less and less attention was given to the "whole" patient and more and more to the causative agent and the specific means at hand for ridding the host of the invader. This concept finally became the most important aim of the clinician, although it did not fulfill all the requirements of therapy. The objective of complete therapy is not only the removal of the infecting organism; it is also to return the patient to a normal or, more ideally, to an optimal state of health.

In Hippocrates' time, anti-infectious therapy was limited to fortifying the patient with pure water, fresh air, good food, soothing concoctions, and vegetable extracts. At the beginning of the present century, the physician thought in terms of the "magic bullets" of specific chemotherapy, neglecting to some degree the battlefield of infection—the patient himself.

In 1936 Hans Selye began to emphasize the concept of "stress" in medicine. In contradistinction to the doctrine of Pasteurian specificity, more attention was directed toward the concept of the host's "nonspecific" reactions to the diseased state. Thus another requirement of therapy was emphasized. According to Selye, as long as man has used the word "disease" he has unconsciously entertained the notion of "stress." If this single term can designate a whole series of individual dysfunctions, then such dysfunctions must possess a common denominator, i.e., certain "nonspecific" aspects that enable us to differentiate disease from health. Because stress manifestations are not characteristic of a single type of infection, they received relatively less medical attention than specific diseases in recent years. They were considered of little or no help in recognizing the nature of the infection and, in any case, there was no specific therapy for them.

The human organism, according to Selye, responds in a stereotyped fashion to a series of very different conditions: infection, intoxication, shock, nervous tension, heat, cold, muscular fatigue, and radiation. The only thing these have in common is that they plunge the host into a state of generalized nonspecific stress. One of the principal causes of stress is infection, considered in terms not of the specific response of the host to each microbial agent but of its capacity to cause stress and therefore to increase metabolism. This happens in wounds, surgery, shock, and burns.

From time immemorial it has been known that infections lower man's organic defenses and, inversely, that he is most likely to contract infections when organic defenses have been reduced to a minimum. Infection represents an intensified form of life in which bodily functions are accelerated, causing profound metabolic alterations. Anorexia reduces the patient's food intake, while most of whatever food is ingested is eliminated through perspiration, the urine, and the forced ingestion of fluids that "wash" away water-soluble vitamins indispensable for fighting infection.

Prolonged ingestion of antibiotics causes metabolic disturbances through alteration of the intestinal flora, which, in turn, upsets certain delicate functions of intestinal biology so important for metabolism, such as synthesis of the vitamin B complex. These difficulties in ingestion, absorption, utilization of vitamins, and other nutritional factors, plus anorexia and an increase in the destruction and excretion of food, provoke a situation in which the patient, although well cared for from the etiologic point of view, may well see his *total* nutritional pattern forgotten. It should be noted, however, that for several years now many physicians, without consideration of stress conditions, have been prescribing supplementary vitamins to overcome losses due to alterations in the intestinal flora during antibiotic therapy.

A practical application of the new concept of *stress* is the combined use of antibiotics—such as the tetracyclines and penicillin—and vitamins to combat the vitamin depletion caused by all infections susceptible to the antibacterial action of these drugs. Vitamins strengthen the host against the *stress* caused by infection. Furthermore, they compensate for the deficiency resulting from a prolonged ingestion of antibiotics, which tends to suppress the intestinal bacteria whose metabolic processes implement the daily requirements of vitamin B complex and vitamin K.

From a historical point of view, antibiotics were discovered and used as substances endowed with a *specific* action against certain microorganisms. They fulfilled a need that had existed from the beginning of this century for "magic bullets" against germs. Antibiotics represent the crystallization of the etiologic thinking of Pasteur and Koch at the inception of microbiology. They grew from the philosophic notion that infections not only are of microbial origin but also have an etiologic specificity.

On the other hand, the discovery of vitamins was a great philosophic triumph for the period of positivism that began in the last quarter of the nineteenth century and that had as its greatest exponent Claude Bernard, who, without knowledge of vitamins as such, recognized the importance of maintaining "physiologic balance." It then became of the greatest importance to understand nutrition biochemically, and this materialized in the discovery of vitamins some forty years ago. Until the middle of the nineteenth century, eating was simply a *necessity;* and then it became an *art,* and finally, a *science*—dietetics.

Vitamins entered medicine first as a therapeutic answer to the specific problems of nutritional deficiencies, but later they were incorporated into the art of good eating for the preservation of health. They therefore underwent an evolution similar to that of the antibiotics, which were born as chemotherapeutic agents to treat acute or chronic illnesses and now are used as stimulants for animal development and growth and as food preservatives.

Today, antibiotics are the highest manifestation of modern specific chemotherapy, just as vitamins are exponents of a nonspecific therapy that fulfills an important function in the total pattern of the disease process. The joint administration of vitamins and antibiotics means that after twenty centuries of medicine we can now control *both* the etiologic agent and the disturbed physiology resulting from infection. It is of interest that Pasteur, the greatest exponent of the germ theory of disease, recognized the importance of the profound effect of the infection on the host when he said, *"Le germe n'est rien; c'est le terrain qui est tout."* (The germ is nothing; it is the terrain that is everything.)

Medicine, which for more than two thousand years—from Hippocrates to Pasteur—has tried to strengthen the organic defenses as the best way to fight disease and which since Pasteur has been concerned mainly with the treatment of the etiologic cause of disease, has now completed the cycle and is again concerned with the patient as a person.

The joint use of antibiotics and vitamins, as I point out elsewhere,[1] represents a restoration of the concept that the *whole* patient should be treated, including his nutrition and his psyche, even in the case of infections.

Medicine is *una et indivisibilis.*

ON THE ART OF TRANSLATION AND THE SCIENCE OF ANTIBIOTICS

*t*o punish man for his presumptuous attempt to reach Heaven through the Tower of Babel, the Lord created the confusion of languages so that man might not understand his fellow man. And to redeem man from this Biblical curse, the art of translation was invented. Yet the task of the translator is an inglorious one, for it has been said that to translate is to betray: *"Traduttore, traditore."*

In chapter LXII of the second part of *Don Quixote,* Cervantes relates how his hero, then in Barcelona, enters a house over whose door was written, "in very large letters," the legend "BOOKS PRINTED HERE." The ingenious hidalgo watches them "drawing sheets in one place, correcting in another, setting up type here, revising there. . . ." And then he comes upon a man of prepossessing appearance and solemn mien who translates from Italian into Spanish (Cervantes does not call him a "translator" but an "author," a significant tribute to the creativeness of his task) and addresses him thus: "To translate from one language into another, if it be not from the queens of languages, Greek and Latin, is like looking at Flemish tapestries on the wrong side, for though the figures are visible, they are blurred by the maze of threads that covers them and they do not appear as smooth and bright as on the right side; and translation from easy languages argues neither ingenuity nor command of words any more than transcribing or copying out one document from an-

---

Published in Spanish as the Foreword to *Principios y Practica de la Terapia Antibiotica,* by Henry Welch, Ph.D., Medical Encyclopedia, Inc., 1955.

other. But I do not mean by this to draw the inference that no credit is to be allowed for the work of translating, for a man may employ himself in ways worse and less profitable to himself." And then he adds: "This estimate does not include two famous translators, Doctor Cristóbal de Figueroa in his *Pastor Fido,* and Don Juan de Jáuregui in his *Aminta,* wherein by their felicity they leave it in doubt which is the translation and which the original."

Thus Cervantes joined the legion of those who, through the centuries, have both praised and condemned the glorious and humble task of translation, a task so derided and yet so necessary that without it the only communication between peoples would be the crude dialectic of prehistoric times: the grunt and the cudgel.

Ortega y Gasset said that translating is a "Utopian, humble and exorbitant ambition." In his essay on the fortunes and misfortunes of translation, the great Spanish thinker contrasts the boldness of the writer, who rebels against language and courageously attacks and conquers it, with the timidity and self-effacement of the translator, who never dares flout its authority.

When dealing with technical texts, the translator finds his work relatively easy, since scientific jargon is a cabalistic Esperanto known to specialists all over the world. Its terminology in all languages is woven of threads of similar colors. But alongside that scientific *Volapük* with its universal scope, looms the formidable task of transferring the inherent style and "inner form" of one language into another, of distilling into vessels of new contour the elusive essence contained in foreign languages, which sometimes overlap like two profiles of different color clumsily superimposed by an engraver with unsteady hands.

The work of freeing men from the abyss that separates them—the diversity of languages—may very well be a utopian task, yet it is of world-wide importance. Nature made men different and, to complete —or perhaps begin—her work, she gave them various modes of expression. That is why, as I understand it, the art of translation is a human rebellion against nature and history; for when the translator makes the sounds emitted by the lips of a Zulu witch doctor understandable to the ears of a Park Avenue psychiatrist, he unifies farflung thought. If every language is "a different equation between expression and silence," translation then undertakes the quixotic mission of putting into a given tongue what the latter, by definition, does not say, and thus integrates humanity on a universal scale.

"In the beginning was the Word," says the Bible. In the beginning, the creative word was everything: in a poetic command, it shot flames of light into space, filled the shoreless emptiness with solid things, the huge ocean beds with blue water, the air with polychrome birds, and the earth with plants and animals, and then set man over all. And although the masters of the earth have, unfortunately, used the word to quarrel and become spiritually separated, in the end the word shall prevail. Indeed, it does so already, for there are many on earth who attempt to make of all languages a chamber music recital in which each one plays his own instrument but all tones and sounds are fused into a single universal harmony.

According to Joan Charles, translation was once one of the creative arts, but in our day it is considered a routine very much like transcribing shorthand or copying blueprints. This has inevitably reduced the dignity and standing of the profession. Since it is popularly believed that to be a translator all one needs is an adequate knowledge of the languages involved, the art has lost status and few well-known writers are translators today. For they will not indulge in the luxury of devoting time and talent to a task yielding very little aside from personal satisfaction. A writer who pens a short story for a fashionable magazine earns considerably more than one who translates a good long novel.

As a result of this, translations today leave much to be desired. Rhythm and euphony are as important as the meaning of the phrase translated. A translator can do an author no greater injustice than to translate the author's very personal ideas into mere words. A certain affinity between author and translator is imperative; the translator must be able to project himself into the temperament of the author to be able to preserve the author's personality. The greatest praise we can pay a translator is to negate his translation by saying, "You can't tell that this is a translation." The translator therefore must give up his personal preferences and interpret faithfully those of the author.

Father Ronald Knox, famous for his fiery polemics with the students of Oxford, was already a living legend when ordered by his superiors to retire to a monastery in Shropshire and translate the Bible. Knox obeyed and devoted himself diligently to his task. For nine years he labored, and finally he produced the English version of the Bible, which may one day replace the famous King James version. His critics were numerous, for as Knox himself said, "No one but the greatest scholars would dare translate Saint Thomas Aquinas, but every one, unfortunately, knows how the Bible should be translated."

In his little book *The Trials of a Translator,* Knox wrote of doing what André Gide regretted not having done while he was translating *Hamlet* into French: he jotted down in a notebook his trials and tribulations as a translator, his gigantic perplexities, and the many versions he had made of a single sentence.

Knox tells us what golden rules a translator should follow in his work: he should know well the language from which he is translating, but he should know his own even better; he should always ask himself how a fellow countryman would put the phrase he has translated from the foreign tongue; and he should avoid becoming enslaved to the literal meanings of words. More than a translator, he should be an interpreter, and sometimes use bold paraphrases to interpret the author he is translating. He should also understand the value and danger of archaic turns of speech, and be able to determine whether he should make "up-to-date" translations or not, since, in Knox's words, "to serve meals that meet today's taste almost surely means to bring about tomorrow's indigestion."

In his charming *Letters to a Little Girl,* the great Cuban writer and patriot José Martí speaks to little María Mantilla about the French book *L'Histoire générale,* which he asks the child to translate into Spanish. His words are among the loveliest ever written on the art of translation. The tenderness Martí felt for the child only accentuates the gentleness and depth of his advice: "Translation should be so natural as to make it appear as if the book had been written in the language into which it is translated. . . . In French there are many words which are neither necessary nor graceful (in translation) . . . it would be a good idea for you to read a book written in practical simple Spanish while you are translating—of course, you understand that I do not mean at the very same moment—for then will you have in your ear and in your thoughts the language in which you are writing." He suggests that she read books written in "simple, pure" Spanish full of "meaning and music." The French of the book she is to translate, he tells her, is "concise and direct, as I want the Spanish of your translation to be; you should therefore imitate it as you translate, and try to use the same words except when the French manner of expression—when the French phrase is different in Spanish," so that "the book will not remain, like so many other translated works, in the same strange language from which it comes." When Martí recommends that the girl write on "paper with a good margin, noble and clean," he is describing the pages of his own immortal letter, a Bible for the good translator and a gospel of fine writing.

The grammatical problems of interpretation-translation are overwhelming. English has a much richer vocabulary than Spanish because of its greater capacity to absorb words from other languages. An English-speaking farmer has a range of two thousand five hundred words; an ordinary novel will use about five thousand words, or five hundred less than the King James version of the Bible, three thousand less than Milton, and incomparably less than Shakespeare, whose range was fifteen thousand.

MEN, MOLDS, AND HISTORY

If Spanish appears to be a rich language with only three genders, what then of the Bantu languages of Africa, which have two dozen genders? A Spanish thinker tells us that there are thirty-three words in Eise to express the motion of walking. In Arabic there are five thousand seven hundred fourteen nouns for camel, the emperor of the desert. And since translation does not mean bringing the author to the language of the reader, but bringing the reader to the language of the author, the difficulty increases.

There is no doubt that translation is a most tempting art, but it is also the most difficult. From time immemorial it has been a godsend to exiled intellectuals, from Castelar to Martí, from Toller to Rolland.

"Translation," Marañón said in his prologue to his translation of *El Empecinado,* "is an exercise traditionally associated with the restlessness of the exile and the prisoner. More than anything else, it helps to alleviate the torment of such predicaments. Translation is compatible with a paralyzing stupor of the imagination (brought on by those situations) even when the translation is, as many think, a banal undertaking. Very much like a delicate piece of surgery, or a clever sleight-of-hand trick, translation consists of extracting ideas from the original and grafting them on to the new language while they are still throbbing with life. Of course, the operation may be done crudely because the idea is a tough fruit that can survive anything; but if it is to be done with finesse and precision—qualities which are not always compatible, of course—it requires superlative dexterity and a noble effort which, to the brain behind it, is tantamount to the creative art. Add to this the immense satisfaction the translator feels, many times subconsciously, of doing a service to his native language, because the latter is the symbol of what is most essential and sacred to our country; it goes with us everywhere and under all circumstances. It is when we are far from our homeland that our duty to serve it becomes a pleasurable task or even a religious observance. And even then we do not take into account that very often the émigré or the prisoner depends on translation for his daily sustenance."

Translation is also the most complex of arts. The boy who, struggling with Caesar's *Commentaries,* translated *"Omnibus repletis, Caesar ivit in Galliam summa diligentia"* as "With the buses full, Caesar went to Gaul in a coach" will never forget the rapping he got on the knuckles. Nor will another student forget the punishment he got for translating *"O tempora, o mores"* as "Oh, times of the Moors!" And what about the wretched translator who turned "Brazil, the matchless country" into "the country without matches?" Another famous translation blunder is the one made by the schoolboy who turned the Latin (Oh hateful, fearful Latin!), *"Aeneas, sedens, clavum regit"* (Aeneas, seated, rules the laborer) into "Aeneas, seated on a nail, is enraged."

It is at the price of such mistakes that we evolved from the primitive fear of being scattered all over the face of the earth, which made men build the Tower of Babel, to a certain linguistic unity.

The word "Babel," Ortega y Gasset reminds us, meant "God's door" to some, but to Schiller it was an onomatopoetic word imitating the sounds of a strange language we do not understand—"Babel" stems from the Greek word *barbarízo,* the Latin *balbutire,* the French *babil,* and the Spanish *balbucir.* Translators who labor to make peoples of different languages understand one another have destroyed the Tower of Babel and the myth of the confusion of languages. With their gift of speech in several tongues, they generously offer the world a lay Pentecost of souls and languages.

But now let us turn from translation in general to a specific translation, the one I have had the honor of making of Dr. Henry Welch's book, *Principles and Practice of Antibiotic Therapy.*

ON THE ENDEAVORS AND ACHIEVEMENTS OF THE AUTHOR OF THIS BOOK

It is my good fortune to be a friend and professional associate of Dr. Henry Welch, who is Director of the Division of Antibiotics of the United States Department of Health, Education, and Welfare, and also the editor-in-chief of two journals—*Antibiotics & Chemotherapy,* which is devoted to reporting laboratory and experimental work done in chemotherapeutics, hormones, and antibiotics, and *Antibiotic Medicine,* * which attempts to depict the vast mural of antibiotic therapy as applied by the modern physician in the clinic.

Dr. Henry Welch's life is one of hard work and accomplishment. The best years of Dr. Welch's life are indissolubly linked with the discovery and widespread use of antibiotics; his work and genius have contributed to the making of living history—the history of antibiotics, the most important chapter in all of modern medicine.

Dr. Welch is a man of science in the fullest sense of the term. We do not speak of the honors bestowed upon him, which circle his brow like a laurel wreath, but of his contributions, which keep growing in length and breadth all the time. He is a man of science because, besides having greatly contributed to the progress of antibiotic medicine in the laboratory and the clinic, he is an admirable organizer, constantly working to make of antibiotics not only the medicine of the present but also that of the future, by guaranteeing ever-widening avenues along which antibiotic research may proceed smoothly.

---

* Now entitled *Antibiotic Medicine & Clinical Therapy.*

In the furrows of this book, Dr. Welch has sown a large and fertile portion of the seed of his knowledge. He wrote this book, in collaboration with several eminent scientific authorities of this nation, by dipping his pen into the ink of his own and his associates' scientific experience. His language is terse and succinct. Faithful to Goethe's last cry for "light, more light," Dr. Welch has sacrificed everything else to a clear style that reflects clear thinking.

This book is today a clinical breviary for the physician in his daily practice, just as it will one day be a textbook prescribed by professors of antibiotic medicine—for three years now I have been urging in vain that such professorships be established—who no doubt will exist in the near future to instruct medical students in the most important scientific discipline of our day.

The translation of this book was a labor of love. I have been responsible for thousands of translations in my time, but only a few have I done with deep pleasure. One was *Zurbarán,* a little book by my distinguished friend, W. Somerset Maugham; and another is this book. I undertook both at the personal request of the authors, who were aware that in an agitated life like mine there is little time for translation.

I translated *Zurbarán* during a vacation period in Nice, under warm blue skies and facing the *mare nostrum,* that clear Latin sea of gods and heroes. I did the present translation amid the steel and smoke, the dust and cement of Manhattan, between constant telephone calls, and under the pressure of the medical journals that I edit, literary commitments, lectures, conventions, and research. I snatched moments away from urgent duties, rest, and pleasure to help, in my own modest way, in the diffusion of a work I believe will be of great value to the Spanish-speaking physician. If I had waited for the peace of mind and leisure required for such a task, I would never have completed it. I had to make the translation in short, hurried spurts, with the aid of a dictaphone; I had to go over rough copies on trains and planes or while waiting in stations, afraid of the next stage, guilty over what had not yet been done, and trying to make up for any lack of literary brilliance with clarity of expression.

Frequently, I was obliged to use scientific neologisms. In a science like antibiotic medicine, where so much is still to be done, the scientific neologism is as indispensable as it has been in my own chosen field of specialization, psychiatry. Yet in this present instance, the neologism is not a sign of an impoverished language but rather of an expanding, growing one, to be compared only with the growth of the antibiotics themselves, which are quickly enriching the therapeutic arsenal of modern medicine.

Bichat, the great architect of human anatomy, recommended the creation of a "different language" for what he called the "science of organized bodies." The exploration of the unrevealed zones of reality is often guided—as in the case of antibiotics—by the fabulous eye of the electronic microscope, and so requires the use of neologism without which scientific progress is not possible.

The clinic and the laboratory—harmoniously balanced in Dr. Welch's thoughts and words, for although the laboratory is his daily arena, he never forgets that he is ultimately concerned with the patient in the hospital—have contributed an infinite number of new words to the coffers of medical knowledge in this country. These words, as restless as fledglings eager to fly away to new climes, require such translation as will lend new color to their plumage but will not weigh down their wings. This I kept in mind at all times while erecting the structure of this book in Spanish, and I tried to use stones no less polished than those of its original language.

If any scientific work is to be clear and instructive, it must contain some amount of dialectic repetition, which becomes more evident in translation. This I beg the reader to forgive. It is better to be repetitious but precise than concise but confusing. The author, besides being a research scientist, is a teacher, and out of respect for his twofold aim, I have tried to maintain the didactic tone of his work, which stems from his seeking out the truth and teaching it to his pupils.

Dr. Welch has dedicated his life to the study, research, and development of antibiotics. His exacting official duties consume most of his time, for he bears the grave responsibility of guaranteeing that the antibiotics used in this country are of law-prescribed quality. But when he has a free hour, when he is not lecturing or traveling on official business, he retires to his lovely home in Maryland. There, beside a swimming pool of limpid waters, surrounded by scented foliage and birds like feathered water colors, and attended by his charming family, Dr. Welch, a stately man as majestic-looking as a Michelangelo figure, thinks, writes, and studies, for the subject of antibiotics is the root and substance of his life. From these hours of quiet meditation have come many of the finest pages of his book, many of those carefully thought out, sincere, and courageous studies that have taught thousands of physicians how to use antibiotics, and, above all, how to search for scientific truth and face it like a good bullfighter faces his bull, unflinchingly, and to transmit it purely and ardently as a light and a flame.

The history of antibiotics goes back thousands of years, yet its initial chapters have scarcely been written. I have discussed the tremendous impact of antibiotics on clinical medicine, along with its philosophic meanings, on other occasions. Some day in the not too distant future, university chairs of antibiotic medicine will be created and a *corpus magnum* of this already monumental scientific doctrine will take shape. Meanwhile, this book by Dr. Welch, a man who has won his eminent position in science not by the sudden quick leaps of the political acrobat but by the laborious slow climb of the scientific alpinist, is a pedestal for antibiotic medicine. It is like an easel displaying the vast panorama of antibiotic medicine, including not only the "ordinary" clinical histories—that "small change" of the hospitals—which are the subsoil of modern medicine, but also the great clinical problems and philosophic evaluations of antibiotic medicine that are the heavenly constellations guiding the clinical vessel of the physician today.

The book is finished, but the task has scarcely begun; for this book ushers into Dr. Welch's scientific life, and into the history of antibiotics, what a brilliant Athenian named Plato called two thousand years ago "the second navigation."

BIBLIOGRAPHY

THE NEXT HALF CENTURY IN ANTIBIOTIC MEDICINE AND ITS
EFFECT ON THE HISTORY OF THE CLINICAL CASE HISTORY

1. ALVAREZ SAINZ DE AJA, E.: Sobre patología de los antibióticos, Medicamenta 21:323, Nov. 20, 1952.

2. ANON.: Over million lives saved, Sc. News Letter 67:373, June 11, 1955.

3. ANON.: The use and abuse of antibiotics (Foreign letters), J.A.M.A. 157: 838, March 5, 1955.

4. CANNAN, R. K.: The cultivation of the improbable; being random thoughts on medical research. Read at the 53d Annual Meeting, Medical Library Association, Washington, D. C., June 15, 1954.

5. CANNON, P. R.: The changing pathologic picture of infection since the introduction of chemotherapy and antibiotics, Bull. New York Acad. Med. 31:87, Feb., 1955.

6. CLARK-KENNEDY, A. E.: The nature of disease, Brit. M.J. 1:473, Feb. 27, 1954.

7. COLLIER, H. O. J.: Chemotherapy of Infections, London, Chapman & Hall, Ltd., 1954.

8. COLLINS, A. J.: Certain aspects of modern drug therapy, M.J. Australia 2:1, July 3, 1954.

9. DALRYMPLE-CHEMPNEYS, W.: Non-specific physiological factors controlling the phenomena of parasitism, Proc. Roy. Soc. Med. 48:13, Jan., 1955.

10. GADDUM, J. H.: Clinical pharmacology, Proc. Roy. Soc. Med. 47:195, March, 1954.

11. GARROD, L. P.: Chemicals versus bacteria, Proc. Roy. Soc. Med. 48:21, Jan., 1955.

12. GREEN, F. H. K.: The clinical evaluation of remedies, Lancet 2:1085, Nov. 27, 1954.

13. HANS, H. B.: Zur Extension der Schrägbrüsche des Oberschenkel Schaftes, München. med. Wchnschr. 96:563, 1954.
14. HIMSWORTH, H.: The integration of medicine, Brit. M.J. 2:217, July 23, 1955.
15. KREBS, H. A.: Excursion into the borderland of biochemistry and philosophy, Bull. Johns Hopkins Hosp. 95:45, July, 1954.
16. LAIN ENTRALGO, P.: La Historia Clínica, Madrid, Consejo Superior de Investigaciones Científicas, 1950.
17. MACKENNA, R. M. B.: The art of dermatology, Brit. M.J. 2:449, Aug, 20, 1955.
18. PAYAN, J.: Science and mankind, Brit. M.J. 2:1415, Dec. 27, 1952.

ANTIBIOTICS TODAY AND THE MEDICINE OF THE FUTURE

1. BERG, H.: Editorial, München. med. Wchnschr. 17:459, 1954.
2. GUTHRIE, D.: Trends and fashions in medicine, Bull. Post-Grad. Comm. Med., Univ. Sydney. 9:209, Sept., 1953.
3. LAIN ENTRALGO, P.: El médico en la historia, Fourteenth Congress of Medicine, Rome, Sept., 1954.
4. LONG, E. R.: The decline of chronic infectious diseases and its social implication, Bull. Hist. Med. 28:368, 1954.
5. MARTI-IBAÑEZ, F.: Historical perspectives of antibiotics: past and present. In: Antibiotics Annual 1953–1954, New York, Medical Encyclopedia, Inc., 1954, p. 3.
6. MARTI-IBAÑEZ, F.: The philosophical impact of antibiotics on clinical medicine. In: Antibiotics Annual 1954–1955, New York, Medical Encyclopedia, Inc., 1955, p. 13. Also in this book, page 9.
7. NOUY, L. DE: Biologic Time, New York, Macmillan Co., 1937.
8. PRATT, R., AND DUFRENOY, J.: Antibiotics, ed. 2, Philadelphia, J. B. Lippincott Co., 1953.
9. SIGERIST, H.: Développement de la médecine préventive, Supp. of Méd. et Hygiène, July, 1954.
10. VALVERDE, M.: Albarrán, Vida Nueva, 1954.

IN QUEST OF THE BROAD SPECTRUM

1. MARTI-IBAÑEZ, F.: The philosophical impact of antibiotics on clinical medicine. In Antibiotics Annual 1954–1955, New York, Medical Encyclopedia, Inc., 1955, p. 13. Also in this book, page 9.
2. WAKSMAN, S.: Definition of antibiotics, Antib. & Chemo. 6:90, February, 1956.
3. MARTI-IBAÑEZ, F.: Antibiotics today and the medicine of the future, Antib. & Chemo. 5(supp. 1):21, April, 1955. Also in this book, page 43.

ANTIBIOTICS AND THE PROBLEM OF MEDICAL COMMUNICATION

1. MARTI-IBAÑEZ, F.: Words and images in medical communication, Internat. Rec. Med. 169:32, January, 1956.

2. MARTI-IBAÑEZ, F.: Books in the physician's life, Internat. Rec. Med. & G.P.C. *168*:650, October, 1955.

WORDS AND RESEARCH

1. LAIN ENTRALGO, P.: España como problema, Madrid, Seminario de Problemas Hispanoamericanos, 1949.
2. SINGER, C.: History and Technology, London, Oxford University Press, 1954.
3. ROF CARBALLO, J.: Segismundo Freud y los problemas de la medicina actual, Bol. d. Inst. Pat. Med. *12*:129, May, 1956.
4. HILDEBRAND, J. H.: Science in the Making, New York, Columbia University Press, 1956.
5. MELICOW, M. M.: Interrelationships of Medicine and Art, Bull. New York Acad. Med. *33*:347, 1957.

ON TREATING THE WHOLE PATIENT

1. MARTI-IBAÑEZ, F.: In quest of the broad spectrum. Some philosophical perspectives of antibiotics, Internat. Rec. Med. & G.P.C. *168*:103, March, 1955.

INDEX

Asclepiades, 14 *n.*
Asepsis, 58
Ataraxics, use of, 71
Auenbrugger, Leopold, 73
Avicenna, 16
  Canon of, 68, 71

Bacon, Francis, 7
Bacon, Roger, 40
Bacteria—*see Microbes*
Bacteriology, history of, 57–58
Beethoven, Ludwig von, 89
Berg, Heinrich, 49
Bernard, Claude, 22, 82, 91, 94, 95
Betts, W. R., 24
Bichat, Marie, 27, 93–94, 103–105
Biggs, Herman T., 78
Biographic concept of disease, 32, 42 *n.*
Bioses, 33
Blegny, Nicholas de, 70
Boerhaave, Hermann, 27, 71
Bouillaud, J. B., 11
Braque, Georges, 85
Bright, Richard, 42 *n.*
Broad-spectrum antibiotics, 57–64

Cancer, 21
Canon of Avicenna, 68, 71
Cardiopathy, 21
Case history—*see Clinical case history*
Castelar y Ripoll, E., 101
Cathastases, 26–27
Cellini, Benvenuto, 71
Cervantes, Saavedra, Miguel de, 97–98
Cézanne, Paul, 85
Chain, Ernst Boris, 1, 73, 90
Chairs of Antibiotic Medicine, 7–8, 22, 40, 41, 78
Charles, Joan, 99
Chemistry, antibiotics and study of, 17
Chemotherapy, antibiotics and, 93, 96
  origin of, 58, 59
Chesterton, Gilbert Keith, 16
Chirico, Giorgio de, 85
Cicero, 83

Clinical case history, antibiotics and, 25–42
  defined, 26
  development of, 26–28
  disease and, 29, 31–34, 42 *n.*
  educational value of, 39–42
  environment and, 29, 37–39
  features of current, 28–29, 42 *n.*
  importance of, 25–26
  integrating factors of, 29
  microbes and, 29, 34–36
  patients and, 29–31
Clinical experimentation, antibiotics and, 21–22
Clinical medicine, antibiotics and, 9–24, 49–50, 53 *n.*–54 *n.*, 63–64
  see also Medicine
Clinical studies, laboratory diagnoses and, 5–6
Communication—*see Medical communication*
Consilium, 27
Corpus Hippocraticum, 68–69, 71

Dale, Sir Henry, 17 *n.*, 62
Dali, Salvador, 85
Darwin, Charles, 91
Data, research and, 83–84
Diagnosis, antibiotics and, 5–6, 60–61
Disease(s), antibiotics and, 12–14, 53 *n.*–54 *n.*
  clinical case history and, 29, 31–34, 42 *n.*
  description of, 82
  environment and, 48
  etiology of, 82–83
  in future, 31–34, 37–39
  as a generic process, 14–16
  natural history of, 20–21
  nature of, 13–14, 31–34, 42 *n.*, 93–94
  philosophy of, 12–14, 31–34, 42 *n.*
  treatment of, 11, 14–16
Disinfection, 58
Domagk, Gerhard, 30, 58, 93
Dosage of drugs, 19
Dubos, René Jules, 1, 42 *n.*, 54 *n.*
Dufrénoy, J., 54 *n.*

112

Quastel, J. H., 17 *n.*
Quinine, 59

Raistrick, H., 90
Ramón y Cajal, S., 1, 74, 91
Rehabilitation, antibiotics and, 50
Rembrandt, 89
Research: on antibiotics, background of, 66–68
  data and, 83–84
  industry and, 84–85
  words and, 79–87
Resistance of bacteria to drugs, 16–17
Rocky Mountain fever, 54 *n.*
Roentgen, Wilhelm, 73
Rof Carballo, J., 82
Rolland, Romain, 101
Russell, Bertrand, 42 *n.*

Salvarsan, 58
Science, language of, 52–53
Scleroses, 33
Search for data, 83–84
Selye, Hans, 10, 31, 94
Semantics, 75–76
Semmelweis, Ignaz, 57, 58
Serums, 36
Servet, Miguel, 8, 73
Seurat, Georges, 85
Singer, C., 81
Smallpox, 20, 36
Soil, antibiosis of, 3–4
Species morbosa, 53 *n.*
Spinoza, Baruch, 87
"Stress" in medicine, 94–95
Sulfonamides, gonorrhea and, 17
  introduction of, 58, 59
Surgery, antibiotics and, 19–20, 54 *n.*
  in future, 38
Sydenham, Thomas, 32, 75
  clinical case histories of, 27, 29
  on disease, 12–13, 82 *n.*
Symbiotic bacteria, 57
Symbols, 75–76
Syphilis, 20, 54 *n.,* 59, 60

Tanguy, Y., 85
Tauer, C. C., 42 *n.*
Teaching—*see Medical teaching*
Team work, individual work and, 2

Technology, words and, 80–81
Tetanus, 36
Tetracyclines, facets of, 61–63
Therapy, antibiotics and, 61
  changes in, 2
  in future, 38
  simplification of antimicrobial, 61
  of whole patient, 15, 93–96
Thompson, George, 37
Toller, Ernst, 101
Tonsillar pseudomembrane, 61
Toxicity of antibiotics, 4, 16, 53 *n.–* 54 *n.*
Translation, difficulties of, 97–102
  of *Principles and Practice of Antibiotic Therapy,* 102–105
Treatises of Galen, 68, 71
Treatment—*see Therapy*
Tuberculosis, 54 *n.*
Tyndall, John, 2
Typhoid fever, 21, 60

United States, antibiotic journals in, 7
Universality of antibiotics, 3–4
Urology, antibiotics and, 20

Vaccines, 36
Vergil, 91
Vesalius, Andreas, 26, 27, 67
Virchow, Rudolf, 53 *n.,* 82
Vitamins, importance of, 95–96
  misuse of, 21
Vuillemin, J., 12

Waksman, Selman, 1
Wassermann's reaction in syphilis, 61
Weizsäcker, V. von, 33
Welch, Henry, in tribute, 102–105
Widal's reaction in typhoid, 61
Woods, 17 *n.*
Words, humanity and, 87
  knowledge and, 86
  medicine and, 80
  pathology and, 81–83
  research and, 79–87
  technology and, 80–81
World Health Organization, international campaigns of, 3
Writing, art of clear, 73–75

ABOUT THE AUTHOR

Born in Cartagena, Spain, Dr. Félix Martí-Ibáñez studied at the Medical School of the University of Barcelona and received his Doctorate in Medicine from the Medical School of the University of Madrid. From 1931 to 1939 he practiced psychiatry in Barcelona and lectured throughout Spain on psychology, medical history, eugenics, art, and literature. During this period, he also edited several medical and literary journals and wrote two novels as well as several books on the history of medicine and psychology.

In 1937 Dr. Martí-Ibáñez was appointed General Director of Public Health and Social Services of Catalonia, and later, Under-Secretary of Public Health and Social Service for Spain. He officially represented Spain in 1938 at the World Peace Congresses held in Geneva, New York, and Mexico City. Upon his return to Spain, while serving as a Major in the Medical Corps of the Spanish Air Force, he was wounded.

After his arrival in the United States in 1939, Dr. Martí-Ibáñez held positions as Medical Director with three leading pharmaceutical concerns. He has lectured in many Latin American universities and has participated in the International Congresses of History of Medicine, History of Science, Psychology and Psychiatry, held since 1950 in Amsterdam, Paris, Stockholm, Nice, and Zurich.

MD Medical Newsmagazine, of which Dr. Martí-Ibáñez is the Editor-in-Chief and publisher, was launched by him in January, 1957. He is the Editor-in-Chief of the *International Record of Medicine;* International Editor of the *Journal of Clinical & Experimental Psychopathology;* and Associate Editor of the two journals he created with Dr. Henry Welch, *Antibiotics & Chemotherapy* and *Antibiotic Medicine & Clinical Therapy.* He and Dr. Welch also founded the Annual Symposia on Antibiotics.

The New York Medical College, Flower and Fifth Avenue Hospitals, appointed Dr. Martí-Ibáñez Professor and Director of the Department of the History of Medicine in 1956.

The Order of Carlos J. Finlay was presented to Dr. Martí-Ibáñez in 1955 by the National Academy of Sciences of Cuba and by decree of the Government of Cuba in recognition of his scientific and educational work in medicine. Recently he was made honorary member of the Turkish Society for the History of Medicine, The Society of the History of Medicine of Brazil, and the Cuban Society of the History of Medicine. He is also a member of fifteen American and European medical, historical, and literary associations.

Medicohistorical and scientific papers by Dr. Martí-Ibáñez have been published in journals throughout the world. Some of his articles and short stories have appeared in *Town and Country, Esquire, Gentry, Art & Architecture,* and fantasy story magazines, and he is also a regular contributor of columns to Latin American newspapers and magazines. Dr. Martí-Ibáñez is now engaged in writing a tetralogy on the history of medicine: the first two books in this series, *Centaur: Essays on the History of Medical Ideas* and *Men, Molds, and History,* were published in the fall of 1958. The other two, *The Fabric of Medicine* and *An Outline of Medical History,* will appear in 1959.

A NOTE ON THE TYPE AND DESIGN

The text of this book has been set on the Linotype in a type face called Times Roman, derived from Times New Roman, which was designed in 1932 for the newspaper The Times of London by Stanley Morison, the well-known typographic adviser to the Monotype Corporation, Ltd. This design was cut simultaneously by both the English Linotype and Monotype Companies as an interchangeable face.

The chapter titles in this book are set in a type face called Lydian, an original design cut by Warren Chappell and first issued by the American Type Founders in 1938.

The initial letter of each chapter is in the American Uncial type face, designed by Victor Hammer, distinguished American artist and typographer. The result of thirty years of study and experimentation, American Uncial is derived from German Uncial.

This book was composed, printed, and bound by The Colonial Press Inc., Clinton, Massachusetts.

The typography, binding, and jacket designs are by Ted Bergman.